T0265916

ADVANCE PRAISE

"I admire how Dr. Mercola has committed his career to pursuing the root causes of what ails us in the modern world, and *Your Guide to Cellular Health* does just this. The book gave me several novel ideas to think about in regard to the metabolic crisis occurring in our cells, and is a useful resource for those seeking to explore new dimensions about how our cells are struggling (and how to support them) in this modern, increasingly toxic world."

> —**Dr. Casey Means,** MD, #1 *New York Times* best-selling author of *Good Energy*

"Demonstrating well-earned lifetime mastery of the subject of holistic health, Dr. Mercola has penned what may be the most revolutionary medical and health text of the modern era. His book masterfully reframes the quest for human health, longevity, and joy with an advanced, holistic understanding of the human experience at all levels—physical, biochemical, and spiritual. It is no exaggeration to say that Dr. Mercola's writings render much of the modern medical establishment utterly obsolete. Even more, his seminal work promises to unleash a new era of spontaneous healing that transcends the models of sickness and disease 'treatment,' once and for all unleashing a paradigm of authentic, sustainable, and reproducible healing through regenerative processes that have been deliberately suppressed by the pharmaceutical cartels. Speaking with a bold voice from a place of endearing courage, Dr. Mercola's book *Your Guide to Cellular Health* should be required reading for all practitioners in the healing arts, and I believe it will one day be recognized as a transformative turning point in the history of medicine. Dr. Mercola is to be widely applauded for this masterful work, and our world is much better off as a result of his effort."

> —**Mike Adams,** a.k.a. The Health Ranger

"Dr. Mercola has spent a lifetime seeking answers on what exactly is a healthy lifestyle. He seeks a scientific explanation for what works and what doesn't work, and he often uses himself as a guinea pig to evaluate different strategies. If you are familiar with his former views on diet, you will be surprised to see his newfound enthusiasm for a high-carb diet that threads throughout this book. I wholeheartedly agree with him that mitochondrial health is essential for cellular health, which in turn is a prelude to vitality, well-being, and longevity. This book reveals a brilliant mind determined to understand how biology works and how it gets derailed by toxic exposures and nutritional missteps in the modern world. It should be essential reading for all those who care about long-term health and well-being."

—**Stephanie Seneff**, senior research scientist, MIT Computer Science and Artificial Intelligence Laboratory

"Dr. Mercola has unraveled the mystery of how to reverse the damage from consuming processed foods, damaging your gut, and running your mitochondria underpowered for most of your life. You would have to read tens of thousands of scientific papers, like I do, to get this valuable information anywhere else, let alone in one concise volume, with actionable items. I highly recommend not only reading this book but adopting as many of the suggestions as possible."

—**James Clement**, JD, LLM, PhD, president and chief scientific officer, Betterhumans Inc.

"This book is more of a detailed textbook treatise of information written in a most informative format quite useful to laypeople and professionals (including me) alike. I like the book—a lot! I am personally a vegetarian, eating and benefiting long term from Dr. Mercola's last step in his reprogramming of the gut, but absent flesh and eggs, and still enjoying excellent health. The book is terrific for the nonvegetarian challenged with gut, energy, and chronic health issues, addressing well the fundamental causes of why your metabolic and digestive processes may be deficient. I heartily endorse the book for both laypeople and professionals. Our so-called disease maintenance 'Health Czars' would also do well to read this amazingly well-referenced 'encyclopedia of health.'"

—**Robert Jay Rowen**, MD

"Dr. Mercola's new book, *Your Guide to Cellular Health*, is just what you would expect from the man who has been on the forefront of medical science and research for the last thirty years. Diseases can neither be cured nor prevented unless the causes are known and treated. And while pharma-based medicine has been busy developing more and more expensive and dangerous drugs that do nothing to address these causes, Dr. Mercola has brilliantly presented the ultimate reason we get sick and die prematurely—it's poor mitochondrial function. And where does that start? Mercola presents an excellent case that the genesis of poor mitochondrial function and hence all disease starts in the intestines with an imbalance of our intestinal bacteria. He also lists the factors that lead to this imbalance, opening the path to longevity and joy!"

—**Frank Shallenberger**, HMD, MD, ABAAM, FAAO, author, editor, researcher, and physician

"I have practiced medicine for over thirty years. One of the most important things I have learned is to identify the underlying cause of an illness. Only then can a proper treatment plan be implemented. The number one complaint I hear from my patients is that they are fatigued. America is exhausted. The vast majority of patients feels like their energy levels are depleted. Dr. Mercola's book *Your Guide to Cellular Health: Unlocking the Science of Longevity and Joy* identifies the root causes of fatigue and provides a pathway for patients to get their energy back.

"The mitochondria are our powerhouse cells responsible for producing the energy molecules—ATP—that fuel the body. For many, mitochondrial dysfunction is at the root cause of fatigue. Dr. Mercola lays out a twelve-step holistic plan to restore the health to our mitochondria and how to maintain mitochondrial health.

"Healthy mitochondria can produce all the energy we need. Fatigue can be overcome through a holistic lifestyle. *Your Guide to Cellular Health: Unlocking the Science of Longevity and Joy* provides the plan for achieving your optimal health. This book is a must-read for those suffering from fatigue."

   —Dr. David Brownstein

"Dr. Mercola's new book has targeted the most fundamental aspects of health and longevity, which are cellular function and energy production. This book gives an actionable and stepwise plan for improving your health from the ground up. Mercola also covers the harm of a lot of environmental factors that could undermine our long-term health. No matter your level of knowledge about nutrition, exercise, or longevity, everyone can learn something new and valuable from this book."

   —Siim Land, author of *Metabolic Autophagy* and expert in intermittent fasting and biohacking

"Dr. Mercola has spent his lifetime as a healer, researcher, and teacher. He is not scared to take on difficult issues and confront them head-on. With his new book he has cracked the code for eternal health. He challenges many conventional wisdoms. In particular, his insights into the populations of bacteria that make up our microbiome are fascinating and revolutionary. A better understanding of one's microbiome will lead to better health. This book should be required reading for medical students and practicing physicians alike."

   —Paul Marik, MD, FCCM, FCCP

"I just read Dr. Mercola's new book, *Your Guide to Cellular Health*. This is a must-read for people who have failure to thrive, which now is a *very* large percentage of the population. The Chinese have said for more than a thousand years that disease starts in the gut. I believe Joe has proven that Chinese statement quite convincingly in *Your Guide to Cellular Health* and has detailed how to fairly quickly reverse many health challenges. The information in this book is simple enough to understand and implement so that almost everyone should be able to benefit. Dr. Mercola has more than two thousand peer-reviewed references from the medical literature to back up his statements and conclusions. Please do yourself a favor, if you have any unresolved health challenges, read *Your Guide to Cellular Health* and apply Dr. Mercola's suggestions to see if you can overcome them with these easy-to-follow words of his advice."

—**W. Lee Cowden**, MD, MD(H)

"'The measure of intelligence is the ability to change.' We must be able to adapt and modify our strategies as new information about our health is available. This sentiment perfectly encapsulates Dr. Joseph Mercola's approach in his latest book, where he once again demonstrates his profound knowledge of health and wellness. Offering a unique and forward-thinking perspective, Dr. Mercola sets himself apart with his ability to adapt and integrate new information, presenting a singular concept aimed at improving overall well-being.

"His recommendations often precede mainstream acceptance, highlighting his role as a pioneer in health. Dr. Mercola's ability to distill complex topics into actionable advice makes this book not only informative but also practical for readers eager to enhance their health.

"His insights continue to lead the way, offering readers valuable tools for navigating the ever-evolving landscape of health and wellness. This book is a must-read for anyone looking to stay ahead of the curve and embrace a healthier lifestyle."

—**Dr. Jason Sonners**, PhD, DC

"Dr. Mercola continues to bring cutting-edge and practical information about healthy cellular function that you just can't find anywhere else. He presents the science clearly to anyone who is inspired to improve their health and energy levels. With so many chronic health epidemics, we need this now, more than ever before."

—**Peter Sullivan**, founder and CEO, Clear Light Ventures, and environmental health advocate

"Dr. Joe Mercola's *Your Guide to Cellular Health* merges a unique vision and bold innovation, offering a revolutionary understanding of the root causes of illness through the lens of cellular mechanisms. His work not only promises a pathway to extended life and enhanced joy but also marks him as a courageous pioneer at the forefront of health science."

—**Dr. Yoshi Rahm**, MD

"Dr. Mercola has been a resource for me since 2008, when I began searching for information to help patients become healthier beyond the drug pushing that was the mainstay of my educational indoctrination. His website, newsletters, and books have been invaluable resources through the past sixteen years. This book is the pinnacle of Dr. Mercola's wisdom, research, and ability to convey complex issues to the public. *Your Guide to Cellular Health* is a valuable work that will help many people regain and maintain their vitality, because it is packed with not only reasoning but also real-life solutions and step-by-step advice for your process of harnessing energy from the food and environment. You will be pleasantly surprised by the fact that so many delightful foods that were once villainized are now known to be necessary for strength."

—**Dr. Suzanne Humphries**, MD FACP, FASN. Co-author of *Dissolving Illusions: Disease, Vaccines, and the Forgotten History*

"Being willing to question a paradigm one has deeply invested themselves in is a rare sign of intelligence. Here, Dr. Mercola shares the critical insights he ultimately arrived at after decades of studying the most important question in medicine—what is behind the epidemic of chronic illness that has emerged over the last century?"

—A **Midwestern Doctor**, board-certified physician and author of *The Forgotten Side of Medicine*

"The new book that Dr. Mercola just wrote I consider his most important work to date. He has put together the evolution of his forty-plus years' learning into a guide people can use to understand and treat the root issues that are underneath all health problems to take us back to optimal health. I also have been practicing over forty years and have adopted with my patients these same principles and can tell you they work. Almost no one, and certainly almost no doctors, understand this information and are only treating the effects of deranged metabolism using drugs, which at times may be necessary in severe emergencies but do nothing to address the underlying issues. With the new tests he is developing to assess mitochondrial and gut-microbiome health and the new tools we now have available, a new revolution in health care will come about as more people and doctors are educated on what to do. I cannot recommend enough the importance of everyone reading and embracing these principles in their own lives and am so happy that he brought this book forth now at a time when it is so needed."

—**Kirby R. Hotchner**, DO

"Mercola tells us a fascinating, even exciting, tale of heroes and villains in the world of mitochondria, energy, and the gut biome. His narrative writing style is clear, concise, and easy to follow. The book is an invaluable conceptual contribution to our understanding of the workings of optimal health and provides a practical guide to resolving its modern-day compromises. If you like mysteries, especially with potentially good endings, you surely won't put this one down."

—**Peter M. Litchfield**, PhD, CEO, Better Physiology, Ltd.

"Dr. Joseph Mercola has been one of the greatest influences on my own personal journey in health optimization. I would estimate that he averages being about ten years ahead of others when it comes to predicting health trends and discovering important concepts that nobody else is talking about, well before the rest of the world even becomes aware of major influences on their well-being. Dr. Mercola defies the status quo, is a pioneer for the entire health field, and does robust and thorough research on any topic that he tackles, and ultimately I cannot recommend his work highly enough! He will make his mark in history as one of the most forward thinkers in wellness, biohacking, health span, lifespan, and beyond!"

—**Ben Greenfield**, CEO, Ben Greenfield Life | Co-Founder, Kion

"In a world overflowing with information, Dr. Mercola filters out the noise to highlight the essential and true elements of health. This book simplifies the complex concept of cellular health into straightforward, actionable steps for achieving vitality."

—**Micah Lowe**, founder, Simply O3, and ozone therapy expert

"In this new book, Dr. Mercola again leads the field with his groundbreaking work on a unified theory of disease. He continues to be our mentor and innovator in discovering medical truths to improve health for all. As always, even as an expert in metabolism and vital health, I learned tons from this book, which will enlighten any reader who ventures to know about his body and physiology and how to thrive in this toxic world. Bravo, Dr. Mercola. This is a monumental achievement."

—**David I. Minkoff**, MD

"*Your Guide to Cellular Health* is an empowering guide that unlocks the secrets to vibrant well-being. With a blend of cutting-edge science and actionable advice, Dr. Mercola skillfully explains how cellular energy production is the foundation of health. This book is cutting-edge science that leaves no stone unturned in its quest to help readers achieve peak wellness."

—**Richard Rossi**, founder, daVinci50 Age Reversal Alliance

"Bioenergetics, microbiome, and mitochondria finally coming together, right here in *Your Guide to Cellular Health*. The whole idea of 'it all starts in the gut' becomes very clear with the new understanding of oxygen-adaptive gut bugs. Can't wait to see how this one plays out. With a clear road map and plenty of references, Dr. Mercola has done it again!"

—**Greg Eckel**, ND, MSOM, Energy4Life Centers

"Changing one's perspective is never easy, especially in a field as dominated by tribalism and dogma as health and nutrition. Yet in *Your Guide to Cellular Health*, Dr. Mercola boldly shifts his approach to embrace the bioenergetic model of health popularized by Ray Peat. With this evolution in perspective, he offers readers practical guidance on nutrition and lifestyle choices that can optimize cellular and mitochondrial function for lasting health and well-being."

—**Jay Feldman**, Jay Feldman Wellness

"Humanity is at a crossroads, and we have reached a point where the survival of not just civilization but the human race itself may very well be in danger. Despite massive technological progress, human lifespan, health span, fertility, and intelligence are not only no longer increasing (as they did for most of the nineteenth and twentieth centuries), but have seen striking reversals in the last several decades. These days, rates of chronic degenerative (and often lethal) diseases are not only rising rapidly in all 'developed' countries, but the rates of increase are often the highest in the youngest segments of the population. In other words, our very future is dying . . . assuming it even gets born to start with due to the striking rise in infertility! Colon, lung, liver, and pancreatic cancers considered 'geriatric cancers' just two to three decades ago are now increasingly affecting teens and even children. Obesity, diabetes, heart disease, and neurological diseases (e.g., Alzheimer's disease, Parkinson's disease, Huntington's disease, etc.), which also have traditionally had highly positive correlation with age, are also now decimating even the youngest cohorts. It is becoming clear to even the non–medically trained general public that something in our understanding of health, disease, and life itself is terribly wrong.

"Modern allopathic medicine continues to view the human organism as little more than a clump of mindless and largely inert matter, subject to the inexorable forces of entropy and 'wear and tear,' but that view has clearly led us to a dead end. Yet, if one digs a little deeper into the history of medicine, it quickly becomes clear that an alternative view of health and life not only exists but has been a focus of the careers of some of the most eminent scientists in modern times, many of whom were Nobel laureates (Otto Warburg, Albert Szent-Györgyi, Hans Selye, Ilya Mechnikov, Linus Pauling, etc.). Their views and scientific discoveries paint a strikingly different picture of human life and health. Namely, that the structure of the human organism (our body) cannot be fully understood (let alone healed) without incorporating the concept of cellular energy—the chemical energy produced by our cells from food, with the ultimate source being the electromagnetic energy emitted by the sun. If one cares to look, there is an overwhelming amount of peer-reviewed scientific evidence that cellular energy is the very essence of life. Its abundant and efficient production through an oxygen-dependent process known as oxidative phosphorylation determines not only how 'energetic' we feel, but also controls every aspect of our lives—i.e., our health, our mood, cognition/intelligence, fertility, and even how long we live. Within the framework of bio-energetics—the study of cellular energy production—anything that promotes optimal energy production is ultimately beneficial, and anything that interferes with it is ultimately harmful, and often lethal. Energetic defects quickly become structural defects—a tenet that allopathic medicine continues to vehemently deny to this day.

"Unfortunately, despite the great discoveries by those eminent scientists, their work was viewed with hostility by allopathic medicine, and many of those scientists were ostracized by the scientific community, which ultimately resulted in their work gaining very little traction with the general population. Several attempts have been made throughout the last fifty-plus years to synthesize the ideas of those luminaries and even incorporate those ideas into medical curricula, but such efforts have been both rare and often esoteric or unsuccessful. One of the most concerted and systematic attempts to synthesize (and further expand) the ideas of bioenergetics developed by those luminaries and present them to the general population in more accessible format has been the work of the American biologist/physiologist Dr. Ray Peat. Yet, his work was also viewed by allopathic medicine as either esoteric or unworthy of clinical consideration, while being subjected to relentless censorship and ridicule. That ultimately limited its widespread review and acceptance, just as it did to the work of the luminaries Dr. Peat based his work on.

"The book *Your Guide to Cellular Health* by Dr. Mercola is a strikingly comprehensive, accessible, and actionable synthesis of the work of all those great scientists (including the writings of Dr. Peat) to date, while also adding previously unexplored topics in regards to gut health and our microbiome. Reading just a few pages from the book makes even a non–medically trained person quickly realize that not only has allopathic medicine gotten it (mostly) wrong and thus failed us completely in terms of protecting and improving our health, it may very well have done so deliberately, being almost completely captured by the powerful lobbying and propaganda machines of Big Food, Big Agriculture, Big Pharma, Big Tech, and even Big Government. Worse, with its current severely handicapped approach to both treatment and prevention, and being openly hostile to novel ideas, allopathic medicine is guaranteed to further degrade our health; perhaps even ensure that from birth to death we are nothing more than zombified, sickly, cognitively diminished automatons who are barely surviving and are entirely dependent on a plethora of pharmaceutical drugs that do nothing to actually cure, but only (and at best) mask the symptoms of our ill health. The book *Your Guide to Cellular Health* is a powerful tool against those forces of medical darkness, regardless of whether they stem from ignorance or malice. It not only clearly explains all important aspects of cellular energy production but identifies explicitly the major threats to cellular energy production we all face and offers direct practical solutions/ steps every adult can take to drastically improve their health and either prevent or ameliorate virtually all health conditions. Ironically, many of those conditions are currently considered by medicine to be at best intractable and even incurable. The book will undoubtedly be found appealing by both the general public as well as the more scientifically minded, including medical professionals (assuming they are open-minded enough to read it). For the general public, the book provides clear, concise, and compelling descriptions (including visuals) of most threats we face from our environment and diet, and how they affect energy production, as well as easy and practical solutions/ steps to counter those threats. Unsurprisingly, diet—the direct source of energy for our cells—plays a central role in the book. However, the book also elucidates many other equally important factors influencing energy production that allopathic medicine gets wrong, ignores, or is openly dismissive of, including sunlight, exercise, endocrine disruptors, hormonal factors, social environment, etc. For the health professionals, the book provides detailed technical descriptions of biochemical pathways involved in energy production and an overwhelming number of scientific references corroborating the key role of energy production in our health, as well as the pathogenic role so many environmental and dietary factors have by simply disrupting optimal oxidative metabolism/phosphorylation. Those professionals can easily incorporate the presented scientific knowledge in their daily clinical practice or scientific research.

"All in all, this book is a desperately needed wake-up call for both the general population and the medical profession. It is also a great guide for a change in direction in the health/medical/nutritional fields, and hopefully soon enough will become a reckoning as well for so many false (and even fraudulent) medical dogmas decimating humanity today. Great work and Godspeed!"

—**Georgi Dinkov**, researcher and health consultant

"'How to get more energy' has become a popular topic. Our energy-producing organelles—our mitochondria—generate about 150 pounds of ATP daily when we are in good health. Of course, ATP is used up in milliseconds, which is why we need to produce such large amounts. Yet, many of us suffer from an energy deficit. How can we improve mitochondrial function? Dr. Mercola thoroughly describes numerous methods that not only elevate our energy levels but also improve overall health and significantly reduce the risk of chronic degenerative diseases that plague Americans.

"*Your Guide to Cellular Health* is exceptionally well-researched, grounded in solid science. While occasionally technical, the health improvement strategies are easily comprehensible.

"Let's be realistic: each of us is a unique biochemistry experiment. To achieve optimal health, we should explore the best-supported foods, supplements, exercise, and other approaches, and discover which ones work for us individually. This book provides the tools to do exactly that."

—**Meryl Nass**, MD physician, researcher, writer

"What would your life be like if you had more energy? Dr. Mercola has written an approachable and inspiring deep dive into cellular energy that can help you unlock your full potential."

—**Peter Sullivan,** Clear Light Ventures

The Truth About COVID-19: Exposing the Great Reset, Lockdowns, Vaccine Passports, and the New Normal (2021, with Ronnie Cummins)

EMF*D: 5G, Wi-Fi & Cell Phones: Hidden Harms and How to Protect Yourself (2020)

KetoFast: Rejuvenate Your Health with a Step-by-Step Guide to Timing Your Ketogenic Meals (2019)

Fat for Fuel: A Revolutionary Diet to Combat Cancer, Boost Brain Power, and Increase Your Energy (2017)

Effortless Healing: 9 Simple Ways to Sidestep Illness, Shed Excess Weight, and Help Your Body Fix Itself (2015)

Dark Deception: Discover the Truths About the Benefits of Sunlight Exposure (2008)

Generation XL: Raising Healthy, Intelligent Kids in a High-Tech, Junk-Food World (2007)

Take Control of Your Health (2007, with Dr. Kendra Degen Pearsall)

The Great Bird Flu Hoax: The Truth They Don't Want You to Know About the "Next Big Pandemic" (2006, with Pam Killeen)

Sweet Deception: Why Splenda, NutraSweet, and the FDA May Be Hazardous to Your Health (2006, with Dr. Kendra Degen Pearsall)

The No-Grain Diet: Conquer Carbohydrate Addiction and Stay Slim for Life (2003, with Dr. Alison Rose Levy)

Your Guide to
CELLULAR HEALTH

Unlocking the Science of Longevity and Joy

Dr. Joseph Mercola

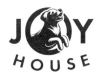

Hardcover ISBN: 978-1-965429-00-6
eBook ISBN: 978-1-965429-01-3

PUBLISHED BY
Joy House Publishing
125 SW 3rd Place, Suite 200
Cape Coral, FL 33991

Joyhousepublishing.com
For rights and permissions please contact media@mercola.com

Book and cover design by Alexia Garaventa

Manufactured in the United States of America

CONTENTS

LIST OF IMAGES

in your gut rise, causing beneficial bacteria to perish while oxygen-tolerant, endotoxin-producing bacteria thrive.

Acknowledgments

The journey of writing this book has been one of discovery, collaboration, and profound gratitude. As we dig into the intricacies of cellular healing, it becomes abundantly clear that we are standing on the shoulders of giants—visionaries whose work has illuminated the path we now tread.

I extend my heartfelt appreciation to all the committed scientists, researchers, and clinicians who have bravely uncovered biological truths and shared them with the world, often in the face of skepticism or opposition from conventional medical models. Their courage and dedication to advancing our understanding of human health have been instrumental in shaping *Your Guide to Cellular Health* and in challenging conventional wisdom to uncover deeper truths about human health.

First and foremost, I must acknowledge the late Ray Peat, PhD, a true giant in the field of bioenergetic theories. His groundbreaking work forms the backbone of much of this book. Peat's tireless efforts to compile and interpret complex biological data have provided an invaluable foundation for *Your Guide to Cellular Health*. His willingness to challenge established norms in pursuit of truth has been a constant source of inspiration.

A special acknowledgment goes to Georgi Dinkov, a Bulgarian IT professional with an extraordinary memory. Georgi has taken up the mantle left by Peat, tirelessly identifying current research that supports and expands upon Peat's bioenergetic approach. His ability to synthesize complex information and draw insightful connections has been invaluable in bridging past theories with present discoveries, further extending the reach of those who came before us.

Ami Ahlstedt deserves profound recognition for her long-standing commitment and invaluable contributions to this project. As the primary chief editor of my newsletter for nearly two decades, Ami brought a wealth of experience and a deep understanding of our mission to the creation of this book. Her agreement to contribute mightily to this project was a game changer.

Together, we formed a formidable team, able to tackle the complexities of the subject matter with efficiency and insight. Ami's dedication, coupled with her editorial expertise, was instrumental in our ability to write this important book in record time, without compromising on quality or depth. Her contributions have been essential in translating complex scientific concepts into accessible, engaging prose.

Ashley Armstrong, PhD, stands as a testament to courage and conviction in the pursuit of health and sustainability. Her decision to transition from electrical engineering to farming, despite financial challenges, exemplifies the kind of paradigm shift needed in our approach to food and health. Armstrong's deep comprehension of Ray Peat's work, which predates my own encounter with it, has been an invaluable resource in refining my comprehension of clinical bioenergetic medicine.

Her vision of transforming industrial agriculture into a regenerative system that truly optimizes our biology is a crucial component of the broader health revolution this book aims to inspire. Her insights and practical experience have greatly enriched the agricultural and nutritional aspects of our work.

Rachel Resnick played a pivotal role in shaping an essential aspect of this book. Her insightful prompting inspired me to articulate the story of my personal hero's journey with my persistent rash. This narrative, which became a powerful thread throughout the book, not only added a personal dimension to our scientific exploration but also served to illustrate the practical applications of our theories. Rachel's encouragement to share this experience has undoubtedly enriched the book's content and its potential to resonate with readers.

Ruth Ann Foster's contribution extended beyond her initial support, proving to be instrumental in refining my personal narrative. Her astute analysis helped identify mercury, rather than oxalates, as the primary culprit in my rash saga. This revelation was not just a personal breakthrough but a testament to the importance of continual questioning and reevaluation in the pursuit of health truths. Ruth Ann's expertise and attention to detail have significantly enhanced the accuracy and impact of this pivotal story.

Kate Hanley, a longtime collaborator who has edited many of my previous books, once again proved her exceptional skill and dedication. Her heroic efforts in providing the primary indispensable edits for this book before it was sent to the developmental editors were invaluable. Kate's keen eye for detail, coupled with her deep understanding of the subject matter, helped to polish the manuscript and ensure clarity and coherence throughout. Her work laid a solid foundation for the subsequent stages of the editing process.

Jessica Sindler, the developmental editor from Kevin Anderson & Associates, brought a new level of structure and flow to the manuscript. Her exceptional job of reorganizing the book's content and putting the pieces in their proper order has significantly enhanced its readability and impact. Jessica's ability to see the big picture while attending to the nuances of each section has resulted in a more cohesive and compelling narrative. Her contributions have been integral in ensuring that the complex ideas presented in the book unfold in a logical and engaging manner for the reader.

Tony Romito's journey with me spans nearly two decades, exemplifying his dedication and growth. Starting in a customer service role and rising to lead our entire content and marketing team, Tony's evolution within the company mirrors the development of our mission. His unwavering commitment, dedication, and selfless service have been truly inspiring.

Tony's overall comprehension of our goals, combined with his innovative approach to content and marketing, have been significant in spreading our message and reaching those who need it most. His contributions extend far beyond his official role, embodying the spirit of our mission in every aspect of his work.

Laura Berry, our CEO, along with the entire executive team at Mercola.com, deserve special recognition for creating the support and infrastructure that have allowed me to serve in a creative role and continue our mission in the most efficient manner possible. Their strategic leadership and operational excellence have been essential in navigating the complex landscape of health information and product development.

Moreover, their efforts to insulate the company from the many attacks hurled at us have been fundamental in allowing us to maintain our focus and integrity. The team's commitment to our mission, coupled with their business acumen, has created a robust platform from which we can continue to challenge conventional wisdom and offer alternative paths to health and wellness.

Arthur Klebanoff's role in bringing this book to fruition cannot be overstated. His expertise and connections in the publishing world were imperative in securing an imprint with Simon & Schuster for our new publishing company, Joy House Publishing. Arthur's guidance in navigating the many challenges of establishing a publishing company was invaluable. His strategic insights and industry knowledge helped us assemble a talented team and put in place the necessary structures to make our publishing venture a success. Arthur's belief in the importance of our message and his tireless efforts to ensure its reach have been fundamental to this project's realization.

I extend my sincere gratitude to Simon & Schuster for their courage and vision in taking a chance on Joy House Publishing as a new imprint. Their willingness to partner with a new publishing company demonstrates their commitment to bringing fresh, important voices to the forefront of health and wellness literature. This collaboration has provided us with a powerful platform to share *Your Guide to Cellular Health* with a wide audience. Simon & Schuster's support, resources, and expertise have been instrumental in bringing this book to publication and ensuring its potential for impact in the field of health and healing.

The 5W Public Relations firm has been an invaluable ally in navigating the complex landscape of mainstream media. Their expertise and extensive network have been essential in addressing past critical articles and effectively communicating our message. Their strategic approach has played a vital role in ensuring that the groundbreaking ideas presented in this book reach a wide audience, overcoming potential barriers and misconceptions. The 5W team's efforts have been instrumental in creating a more balanced narrative around our work, allowing the transformative potential of *Your Guide to Cellular Health* to be considered in the public sphere.

Looking to the future, I want to acknowledge in advance all the Mercola health coaches who will join us in this mission. These individuals will play an all-important role in caring for the readers of this book and aiding them to apply its principles to their daily lives. Akin to the barefoot doctors of the past, these coaches will provide powerful and insightful education, helping people navigate the choices necessary for health recovery amid the noise of propaganda and misinformation.

Their work will be essential in translating the theory presented in this book into practical, personalized health strategies. These coaches represent the front line of our efforts to empower individuals with the knowledge and support needed to take control of their health in meaningful ways.

Without the foundation of love and support provided by my precious parents, this book would never have been possible. Their selfless dedication and unconditional love during my childhood instilled in me an "allergy to fear" that was a building block in my future pursuits. This fearlessness has enabled me to make the brave and courageous choices necessary to create systems that finally allow people access to medical care that addresses the foundational causes of their health challenges. The values they imparted and the nurturing environment they created have been instrumental in shaping not just this book, but my life and entire approach to health and healing.

Lastly, but certainly not least, I must acknowledge my constant companion, Joy—my beloved dog! Joy's unwavering presence (rarely leaving my side) and loyalty has been a source of comfort and stability throughout the writing process. Our daily solar noon walks on the beach have not only provided the physical activity and sun exposure so significant to the theories presented in this book but have also offered necessary moments of reflection and clarity.

Joy's simple, pure presence has been a living reminder of the importance of connection, movement, and natural rhythms in our lives. It's fitting that Joy became the inspiration for my new publishing house, Joy House Publishing, as he embodies the very essence of what this work aims to bring to others—a return to natural, Joyful living. Joy's contribution to this work, while (mostly) silent, has been profound, serving as a constant source of, well, Joy in my life and a living example of the healing power of companionship and nature.

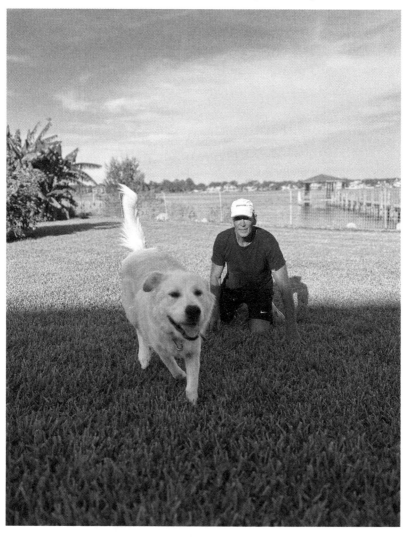

Pawsitive vibes! Enjoying a moment with Joy, my Great Pyrenees puppy.

Note to Readers

The author of this book does not advocate the use of any particular form of health care for all individuals but believes that the facts, figures, and knowledge presented herein should be available to every person concerned with improving his or her state of health. This book is not intended to replace the advice and treatment of the reader's personal physician or health-care provider. Any use of the information set forth herein is entirely at the reader's discretion.

The author and publisher are not responsible for any adverse effects or consequences resulting from the use of any of the preparations or procedures described in this book. This book is based upon the author's own opinion and theories. The reader should always consult with his or her own health-care practitioner before taking any medicine or dietary, nutritional, herbal, or homeopathic supplement, or beginning or stopping any therapy. The author is not intending to provide a substitute for the reader's personal medical advice and makes no warranty whatsoever, expressed or implied, with respect to any product, device, or therapy. No statement in this book has been reviewed or approved by the United States Food and Drug Administration or the Federal Trade Commission. Readers should use their own judgment in consultation with a holistic medical expert or their personal physician or health-care provider for specific applications to their health-care needs.

A Quick-Start Guide to Unlocking Your Cellular Fountain of Youth

CHAPTER 1

Embrace Your Journey to Vibrant Health and Renewed Energy

You have the power to make informed choices about the food you eat and your health. Kimberly's story of overcoming type 2 diabetes by making better choices serves as a beacon of hope and inspiration. By becoming aware of hidden ingredients, you can transform your well-being. The good news is that you can easily avoid harmful seed oils in processed foods. Your body will thank you for this loving act of self-care.

You are already on the path to optimal health by seeking out knowledge. Congratulations on taking this key step! By choosing whole, unprocessed foods, you're nurturing your body's natural vitality. Every healthy choice you make is a victory for your long-term wellness.

Unleash Your Body's Natural Healing Potential

You have the wisdom to see beyond marketing claims and choose truly nourishing foods. By reading labels carefully, you are protecting your precious cellular energy. Trust in your ability to make choices that support your vibrant health. Remember, every small step toward better nutrition is a big win for your well-being.

Celebrate Your Body's Resilience

Your body is incredibly adaptable. Reducing omega-6 fats supports your mitochondria. Embrace the journey back to a more balanced, ancestral way of eating. You have the power to reverse the effects of modern dietary trends and reclaim your vitality.

Empower Yourself with Knowledge

You are becoming a savvy health advocate for yourself and your loved ones. By questioning health claims and researching them, you are in control of your wellness path. Trust your instincts and the power of informed decision-making. Your commitment to understanding health information is admirable and will serve you well in the future.

CHAPTER 2

The Empowering Truth About Reclaiming Your Gut Health

My struggle with a fifteen-year-long stubborn rash catalyzes a major health epiphany. My experience helped me to develop a new theory of health that targets the root causes of disease. It helped me identify the links between cellular energy and gut health. Hidden mercury in my dental fillings and toxic pollutants were the key culprits behind my rash. If you have silver (mercury) fillings, they are harming your health. But, as I learned, having a regular dentist remove them will make you much worse, as they are not trained in the proper safety protocols.

The Dangers of Mercury in Dental Fillings

Dental amalgams contain mercury, a neurotoxic poison that damages your health. Mercury in your fillings causes neurological, immune, and metabolic disorders. Dental amalgams leach mercury into the body over time. They require safe removal by biologic dentists. Detox is helpful to reduce mercury's harm and protect your long-term health.

The Importance of Cellular Energy and Mitochondrial Function

Low cellular energy causes most health problems. Your mitochondria are your cells' energy powerhouses. They generate the power required for all bodily functions. Restoring optimal mitochondrial function improves or resolves most health issues. Specific diet and lifestyle changes rejuvenate your mitochondria. Restoring your mitochondria and gut bacteria to optimal function is the key to unlocking the door to the fountain of youth.

The Connection Between Gut Health and Comprehensive Wellness

My journey taught me that a damaged gut microbiome harms your health. It is vital to keep a healthy gut. This will slow aging, boost your immunity, and prevent most diseases.

CHAPTER 3

Unlock Your Body's Potential for Vibrant Health and Endless Energy

There is a powerful connection between cellular energy and gut health. Low cellular energy is the driving factor behind most health issues. Cellular energy is essential for keeping oxygen levels low in your colon. Excess oxygen in your colon boosts harmful bacteria, which leads to insulin resistance. This imbalance is the underlying cause of many persistent health challenges.

Excess oxygen in your colon harms beneficial bacteria while causing disease-causing bacteria to thrive. This imbalance results in the overproduction of endotoxin, a potent mitochondrial toxin. To restore your health, you must reverse this process. You can do this by nurturing your gut microbiome. A healthy gut is essential if you ever hope to recover your full vitality.

Treating Symptoms, Ignoring the Cause: The Role of Insulin Resistance
Conventional medicine uses expensive new drugs, like Wegovy, to treat obesity and diabetes. It ignores the underlying cause of disease. Insulin resistance plays a significant role in disease. It affects your metabolic health and contributes to most health disorders. The HOMA-IR test is an inexpensive, useful way to easily measure your insulin resistance.

The Fiber and Short-Chain Fatty Acids (SCFAs) Paradox
We detail how fiber is the fuel for your beneficial gut bacteria to produce SCFAs. These fats help keep your gut barrier intact and provide energy to your colon cells to keep oxygen out of your colon. The paradox is that a fiber-rich diet boosts SCFA production, but if your gut is damaged, those "healthy" fibers will feed disease-causing bacteria. These "bad" bacteria will produce endotoxins that destroy your health.

How Environmental Toxins Ruin Your Health
Environmental toxins lower your cellular energy and undermine your gut health. Microplastics and synthetic chemicals are pervasive. They harm your mitochondria. This decreases your cellular energy and increases your risk for most diseases.

CHAPTER 4

Transform Fatigue into Vitality by Tackling the "Four E's" of Cellular Health Risks

There are four major threats to your cellular health. The "four E's" are:

- Excess essential fats (processed vegetable oils)
- Estrogens (including plastic xenoestrogens)
- Electromagnetic fields (EMFs)
- Endotoxins

Vegetable oils in processed foods and even "health" foods harm your cells and cause you to be tired and feel hopeless. Many household products and cosmetics contain endocrine-disrupting chemicals (EDCs). The rise in electromagnetic field exposure from modern tech adds to the problem. All these factors cause harmful gut bacteria to proliferate in your gut. They produce endotoxins and damage your cellular energy. Their combined impact affects your health in ways you never imagined.

Excessive Vegetable Oils Are Fueling the Chronic Disease Epidemic

You likely consume excessive amounts of vegetable oils and seed oils. This lowers your energy and makes you feel tired all the time. Excessive seed-oil consumption is also the main cause of the epidemic of chronic diseases. These include heart disease, obesity, and cancer. They cause leaky gut, neurodegenerative diseases, and heart disease.

The Pervasive Threat of Endocrine-Disrupting Chemicals (EDCs)

EDCs, including bisphenols and phthalates, are common ingredients in plastics and everyday products. Microplastics are pervasive environmental pollutants that accumulate in your body. The average person consumes a credit card's worth of plastic a week. Every year, manufacturers produce half-a-billion tons of plastics. They mimic your hormones and wreak havoc on your endocrine system. EDCs have been linked to reproductive problems, heart disease, cancer, obesity, and diabetes.

Electromagnetic Fields from Your Devices Come at a Cost

Most of us exchange the convenience of our modern devices for health. As a result, electromagnetic field (EMF) exposure has increased dramatically due to modern technology. Chronic exposure to EMFs from devices and wireless networks is toxic to your mitochondria. It lowers your energy and stamina. I provide practical recommendations to help you reduce your EMF exposure.

Harmful Gut Bacteria Lead to a Vicious Cycle of Disease and Premature Death

Impaired energy production in your cells shifts your gut bacteria. It favors disease-causing, oxygen-tolerant ones over beneficial oxygen-intolerant bacteria. This imbalance increases endotoxin production, which is difficult to overcome. It is why almost no one escapes the black-hole spiral of premature death without expert advice.

CHAPTER 5

Let Sunlight Gently Guide and Brighten Your Journey Back to Health

The sun powers all life on Earth. Sufficient appropriate sun exposure is essential to restore and optimize your health. The sun will help your vitamin D, melatonin, and energy production. Its effects benefit your longevity, heart health, and cancer prevention. However, you do need to be cautious with your sun exposure. A balanced approach to sun exposure is key. The right amount of sun will boost your energy and help you recover the health you deserve.

The Sun Alone Does Not Cause Skin Cancer and Premature Wrinkling

Dermatologists are correct; the sun can age your skin and cause skin cancer. What they do not tell you is that it is not caused by the sun alone. Skin cancer happens because the vegetable oils you eat become embedded in your skin cells. The sun then turns them into toxins. Avoid intense sun exposure until you have abstained from vegetable oils and processed foods for at least six months. A sunburn is a sign that you had too much sun exposure for the level of vegetable oils in your tissue.

Unlocking the Power of Vitamin D with Sunlight or Supplements

Sunlight is the best way to produce vitamin D. It is vital for regulating thousands of your genes. Optimal vitamin D levels lower the risk of many diseases. These include cancer, heart disease, and autoimmune disorders. If sunlight is unavailable, most people will benefit from supplementation. Dosing, timing, and other nutrients need to be considered. Vitamin K2 and magnesium will increase the absorption and boost the benefits of oral vitamin D.

Major Benefits of Early Morning and Solar Noon Sun Exposure

Sun exposure, especially in the morning, helps regulate your body's circadian rhythms. Contrast this to solar noon sun, which increases melatonin. Most are unaware that 95 percent of your melatonin is not made in your brain but in your mitochondria. Melatonin destroys free radicals, shielding cells from oxidative harm.

Challenging Misconceptions About Sun Exposure

Not all sun exposure is harmful. It primarily poses risks to those who consume excessive amounts of vegetable oils. Research shows that moderate sun exposure decreases death rates and improves health. To gain health benefits and avoid sun damage, time your exposure and take precautions. The key is to gradually increase sun exposure only after you have eliminated seed oils from your diet for at least six months.

CHAPTER 6

Your Path to Vibrant Health Begins with a Single Step: Discover the Joy of Movement

Movement is a central component of optimal health. A sedentary lifestyle will prevent you from ever fully recovering your health. Benefits of regular exercise include normalizing your insulin sensitivity and hormone balance, and boosting brain function.

Use exercise "sweet spots." Excessive high-intensity workouts are counterproductive. Avoid them. Instead, replace them with moderate activities, such as walking. Walking is one of the best exercises for the whole body. Shoot for one hour of walking, divided up throughout the day.

The Dangers of a Sedentary Lifestyle

Lack of movement causes many health issues. These issues include the deterioration of your muscles and a higher risk of chronic disease. Your body needs frequent regular movement. Sedentary behavior also lowers your energy. It will cause you to die early and suffer needlessly.

Avoid excessive sitting. Standing desks provide an excellent alternate choice for better posture and less back pain.

Exercise Enhances Insulin Sensitivity, Hormones, and Mitochondrial Health

Regular exercise helps your metabolism and increases your energy. It boosts insulin sensitivity, regulates hormones, and supports your mitochondria. Exercise is a powerful tool to help manage your weight, prevent diabetes, and clear your head.

How Exercise Unlocks Your Brain Power

Exercise boosts your brain function and strengthens mental well-being. Regular exercise boosts your BDNF levels. This protein promotes brain growth and survival, and enhances neuroplasticity. BDNF helps your brain adapt, learn, and recover from injury.

CHAPTER 7

Nourish Your Body with Love: Why Embracing Healthy Carbs Can Transform Your Health

Low-carb diets are not healthy in the long term. Carb restriction cripples your cellular energy production. You need balanced carbs for your brain and body health. Long-term low-carb diets release stress hormones and are harmful. When you do not eat enough carbs, your body must create glucose from your muscles. This is dangerous, especially as you age.

There are widespread misconceptions about insulin resistance and carbs. Glucose, not fat, is the optimal fuel for your mitochondria.

Long-Term Carb Restriction Harms Your Metabolism

The long-term benefits of low-carb diets are not well-studied or supported. Over time, a low-carb diet decreases your cellular energy. Prolonged carb restriction is very risky for your health. Most adults need at least 200–350 grams of carbs every day to create enough cellular energy.

Glucose Is Key to Cellular Energy, Health, and Disease Prevention
Mitochondria are vital for your cellular energy and health. You must improve your mitochondrial function to be healthy. Mitochondria make adenosine triphosphate (ATP), the main energy currency for your cells. By efficiently producing ATP, mitochondria are able to fuel most of the work your cells perform.

Your Brain Thrives on Glucose for Energy
Your brain needs a lot of energy. To work well, it relies on glucose as its primary fuel. You must eat enough carbs. It is vital for peak brain performance and mental clarity. Ketones are an alternative fuel, but they do not fully meet the brain's energy needs. Over time, relying on ketones leads to suboptimal brain function.

Focus on Your Gut Health and Tailored Nutrition for Better Energy
Your gut's health and your body's ability to process carbs are closely intertwined. Your microbiome greatly affects how your body metabolizes carbs. Conversely, the types of carbs you eat shapes your gut health. Customizing your approach to carb selection is one of the most important steps in recovering your gut health.

CHAPTER 8

Love Your Cells: How Changing Your Oils Can Rapidly Boost Your Well-Being

The widespread use of vegetable oils has damaged nearly everyone's health. The edible-oil industry led the effort to make these oils common in processed foods. The industry has biased both research and public opinion. They promote these oils as healthy alternatives to traditional fats. It is best to substitute all vegetable oils for traditional fats like butter and tallow. This will help your energy level and weight. One of the most important steps you can take to recover your health is to choose your fat wisely.

The Deceptive Nature of Vegetable Oils
Seed oils, often called "vegetable oils," are highly processed. They

come from crops like soybeans and corn. These oils are in most processed foods. They have long been touted as healthier than traditional fats, like butter and coconut oil. However, harsh chemicals and industrial methods are used in creating these oils. This process creates dangerous metabolic toxins in these oils.

The Importance of Reducing Vegetable Oil Consumption
For optimal health, remove all vegetable oils from your diet. Limit linoleic acid (LA), the main omega-6 fat in vegetable oils, to 5 grams or fewer per day. This means avoiding all processed foods. Choose traditional fats like butter and tallow. Also, be mindful of LA in poultry and pork.

Rethinking "Healthy" Foods
Even "healthy" oils, like olive and avocado oil, will harm your health if eaten to excess. Their high monounsaturated fat content can disrupt your mitochondrial function. It is wise to limit your use of all vegetable and seed oils, including those with a "health halo." Seeds and nuts are also widely considered healthy but are high in LA. Avoid them for six months to lower your LA.

CHAPTER 9

Awaken Your Inner Vitality: How Collagen Can Gently Build and Transform You

Modern diets often lack collagen. Increasing your collagen intake significantly improves your health. Collagen supports cognitive function and longevity. Collagen makes up one-third of your body's protein. It is vital for your skin, bones, and connective tissues. It plays a crucial role in cellular hydration and function.

Glycine, a key component of collagen, extends your lifespan and improves your gut health. Glycine also helps heal wounds, improve sleep, and protect your aging brain. Glycine is not an essential amino acid, as your body makes it, but you cannot make enough to cover your needs. Understanding this helps you make wise choices about using glycine.

You can take glycine supplements, but it is best to get it from whole foods. Gelatin is a type of collagen that is cooked and broken down. Boost your glycine levels by eating collagen-rich foods such as bone broth, or use gelatin or collagen supplements.

It is important to balance muscle meat with collagen-rich foods. There are some dangers in using conventional eggs and cheese. I give guidance for selecting high-quality animal proteins, emphasizing grass-fed and pasture-raised options. There are risks of consuming excess iron and phosphorus from animal proteins. However, there are ways to maintain optimal levels and balance these important minerals.

Consider High-Quality Animal Proteins for Better Health

Protein is required for your muscle mass, immune function, and cellular energy. The quality of animal proteins matters. Choose grass-fed and pasture-raised options when possible, as they have healthier fats. Focus on ruminant animals (ones that chew the cud) like cows, lambs, and goats. Be cautious with non-ruminant proteins like pork and chicken, as even organic versions are fed grains and are high in LA.

Combining Muscle Meat and Collagen Boosts Longevity

Limit your meat intake to a few ounces a day. Eating only muscle meats causes an amino acid imbalance. This leads to excess methionine that decreases longevity and causes thyroid problems. Get one-third of your protein from collagen or its amino acids. This will mimic the protein in whole animals.

Balancing Iron and Phosphorus Intake Is Key to Protecting Your Health and Bone Strength

Excess iron and phosphorus intake from animal proteins are harmful. High iron levels can lead to oxidative stress and chronic health conditions. Excess phosphorus disrupts calcium balance, affecting bone health. It is crucial for optimal health to track and balance these minerals. Do this through diet analysis and supplements.

CHAPTER 10

Your Gut's Rainbow: A Simple Introduction to Carb-Fueled Gut Repair

There are many challenges and myths about carbohydrates. Carbs are vital for your health. They provide energy, support your brain, and help grow muscles. There is a full spectrum of carbs, from simple sugars to complex starches. Each affects your body differently. Easy-to-digest carbs help boost digestion and nutrient absorption.

You need a balanced approach to carbs. It must suit your needs and promote gut healing, not harm it. Unwise carb choices trigger conditions such as SIBO (small intestinal bacterial overgrowth) and candida. Consume carbs with precision targeted toward the current state of your gut health. A novel red, yellow, and green carbohydrate classification provides you with the tools to do that.

Understanding Carbs: From Simple Sugars to Complex Starches

I introduce a novel way to classify carbs. Green is good for everyone. Yellow is something you must progress to. Red is only for those with exceptionally good gut health. This system guides you in picking the best carbs for your current state of health and metabolism. This personalized approach to carb intake allows you to recover your gut health. The best way to improve your gut health is by avoiding carbs that your gut is not ready to tolerate.

Why Low-Carb Diets Fall Short

Many people initially improve on low-carb diets. This is because they reduce fuel for bad bacteria. Not feeding these bacteria lowers endotoxin. However, over time, low-carb diets cause a large drop in your mitochondrial energy and thyroid function. The ultimate solution is to add enough "green" carbs (from the tricolored carb classification chart) to meet your cellular demands. This will increase mitochondrial energy and activate cellular repair and regeneration.

The Fuel Your Brain and Body Can't Live Without

Carbohydrates are your key for energy, brain health, and muscle growth. Most adults need a minimum of 200–250 grams of carbs daily for cellular energy. And half of that is for your brain! Without enough carbs, your cognitive and physical performance will suffer.

CHAPTER 11

Embrace Seven Supplement Solutions to Restore Your Mitochondrial Health

This chapter covers seven key supplements. They can help recover health after exposure to mitochondrial toxins.

- The beneficial oxygen-intolerant bacteria *Akkermansia muciniphila*. Many people have lost significant populations of these bacteria. This is due to decades of poor mitochondrial function. Once you have eliminated mitochondrial poisons, you can add this bacterium as a seed. It is not a "magic bullet" and requires removing mitochondrial poisons discussed in this book. Otherwise, it will not thrive. It will only reproduce efficiently in a healthy colon.

- Most adults benefit from additional progesterone. It counters excess stress hormones and the damage from estrogen-mimicking chemicals.

- Magnesium, low-dose niacinamide, thiamine, calcium, and vitamins D3 and K2 are key nutrients. They target cellular energy depletion from processed foods.

Restoring Gut Health: Why *Akkermansia* Is Essential for a Healthy Microbiome

Akkermansia makes up 3–4 percent of a healthy microbiome. Some experts believe it could be as high as 10 percent. Labs analyzing the human microbiome say that about a third of people have few to no *Akkermansia* at all. This microbe makes short-chain fats that feed and heal your colon's cells. They are essential for you to recover your gut health and regain your energy.

Scientists discovered this bacterium only twenty years ago. There are several companies that have sold this probiotic product over the past few years. They promote their product as pasteurized, which typically implies safety and quality. However, in this case, it means they are killing all the live beneficial bacteria. The first breakthrough product containing live *Akkermansia* will be available in fall 2024.

Progesterone Shields Against Environmental Estrogens and Supports Your Health

Environmental estrogens are practically impossible to avoid. Even if you use glass containers and avoid plastic wraps, some exposure is inevitable. Progesterone counters and even reverses the effects of this constant estrogenic assault on your body. It can also counter high levels of stress hormones, low bone density, and heart and immune issues. Most progesterone is ineffective due to its delivery methods. I provide specific guidance to ensure progesterone absorption is maximized. Synthetic progesterone (progestin) is dangerous and should always be avoided.

CHAPTER 12

Empowering Your Metabolism: A Monthlong Journey to Vibrant Health

Implement my recommendations with this four-week plan. Each week focuses on a different aspect of your lifestyle. It will guide you to unlock your body's potential and energize your metabolism.

> **Week 1: Building Your Foundation for Success.** Get excited about this preparatory week! Choose nourishing foods that align with your goals and improve your gut health. You will discover your unique metabolic rate and calorie needs using simple, at-home tools. This knowledge will help you fuel your body for optimal metabolic performance.

> **Weeks 2 & 3: Embracing Positive Changes.** Celebrate balanced meals and optimized macros during these transformative weeks. Eat moderate protein, especially from collagen-rich sources. Also, eat nourishing fats, such as coconut oil and butter, and energizing carbs. Revel in quicker recovery. Strength training can help. It

builds muscle, boosts metabolism, and improves insulin sensitivity. Enjoy daily, sun-soaked walks to boost your energy and well-being. These walks will also synchronize your body's internal clock, resulting in better sleep.

Week 4: Celebrating Your Progress. In this final week, rejoice! Your gut health and metabolism have improved since week 1. Reintroduce some foods. Fine-tune your body's response. This will create a sustainable, personalized eating plan that works for you.

By the journey's end, you will feel more energetic. You will sleep better and be healthier. Your positive habits will boost your long-term metabolic health. They will ensure continued progress. Congratulations—you're on the path to vibrant health and vitality!

CHAPTER 13

Nurturing Your Cellular Vitality in Today's World

Modern environmental challenges are daunting, but you have the power to make a positive difference. Informed choices in your daily life can reconnect you with nature's wisdom and support your body's innate healing abilities.

Empower yourself with new tools to support your health journey. Try the Mercola Health Coach app and insightful virtual consultations. Remember, every small step you take toward better health is a victory worth celebrating!

Life's Journey—a Tapestry of Choices and Discoveries

Just like all of you, I have had many experiences that have brought me to where I am today. Each step, each decision, each moment of insight has been a thread in the tapestry of my life and career. I am sharing these glimpses into my past with you not just as a personal revelation, but as a mirror through which you might reflect on your own journey.

We often forget that our present awareness is the result of a long and sometimes winding path. The choices we've made, the beliefs we've held, and the knowledge we've gained all contribute to our current perspective on health and wellness. By sharing my story, I hope to illustrate that the journey to optimal health is not always a straight line. It's a path of discovery, often marked by unexpected turns and revelations.

I want you to see these snapshots of my life and then place your own life choices in context. Where are you in your own experience of your biology and health? What beliefs have shaped your journey so far? What moments have been pivotal in your understanding of wellness?

It's important to acknowledge that I did not always make choices that align with what I know now. There were times when I followed conventional wisdom without question, and times when I made decisions based on incomplete information. But these experiences have been invaluable in shaping my current perspective.

This collection of images represents my evolving relationship with health, science, and self-discovery. It's a visual narrative of how one's perspective can change over time, how new information can reshape our worldview, and how the pursuit of knowledge can lead us down unexpected paths.

As you look at these photos and read their captions, I encourage you to reflect on your own journey. Remember, we are all works in progress. My story is still unfolding, as is yours. Let these glimpses into my past serve as a reminder that it's never too late to learn, to grow, and to make choices that align with our deepest perception of health and wellness.

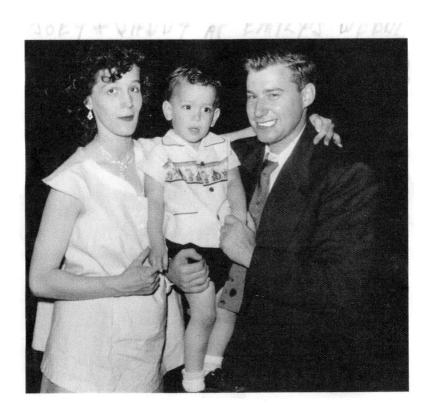

Just shy of two years old, I'm pictured with my pregnant mother and father at the wedding of a family friend. It's a snapshot of family growth and new beginnings that would shape my understanding of the interconnectedness of health and relationships.

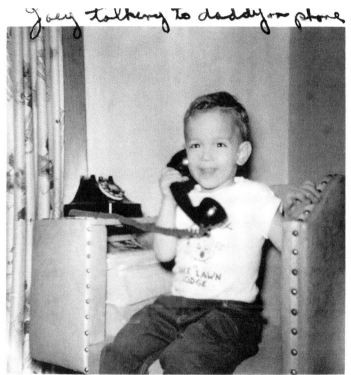

Joey talking to daddy on phone

2 YEARS OLD

At the age of two, I am beaming with Joy as I master the art of conversation (with Dad) on a rotary phone. Even then, the seeds of curiosity, connection, and enthusiasm were being sown, foreshadowing a lifetime of passionate exploration in health and wellness.

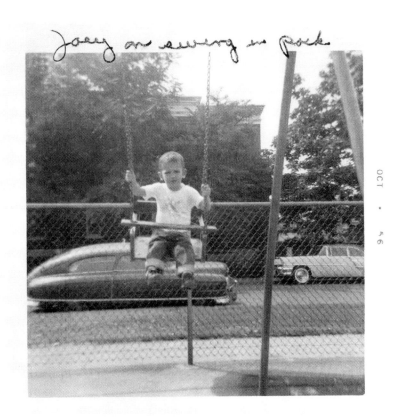

At two years old, I am flying high and carefree on a playground swing. It's a memory of pure Joy that would later help bring awareness to the importance of play and movement in overall health in life.

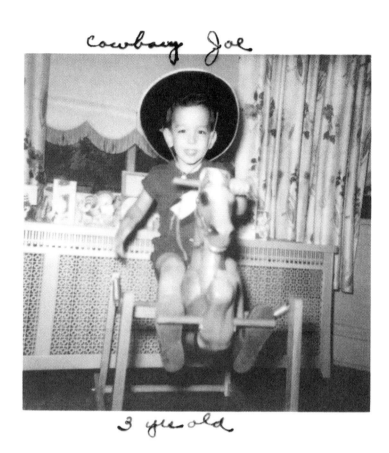

At the age of three, "Cowboy Joe" is ready to ride off into the sunset on his trusty rocking horse. Little did I know that my adventurous spirit would lead me on a lifelong journey down the trail of health discovery.

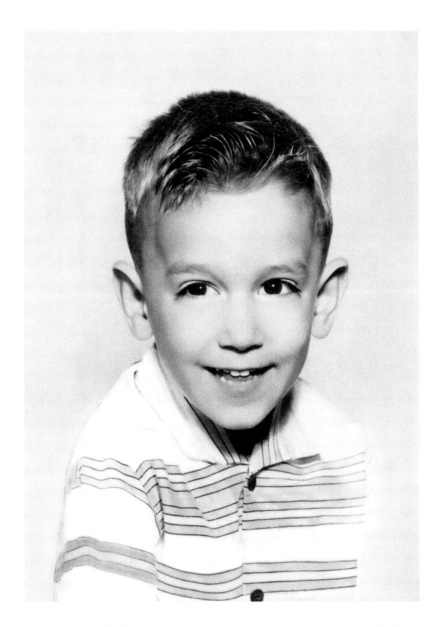

At three years old, I am full of wide-eyed wonder and endless questions. Looking back, those early days of exploration set the stage for a lifetime of learning and discovery.

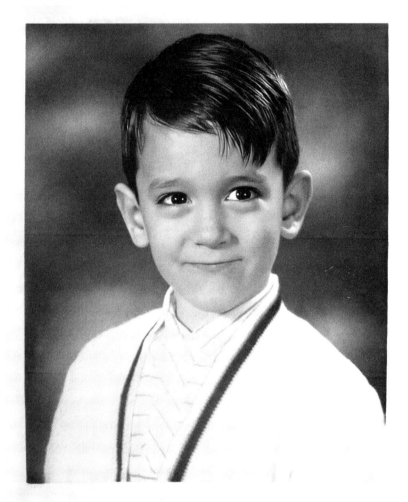

ST. MEL SCHOOL
1959-60

At five years old, I was a proud kindergarten graduate. This early academic milestone marked the beginning of a lifelong passion for learning and understanding the world around me.

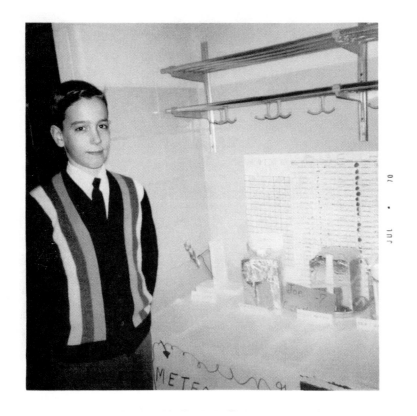

At fourteen years old, I am standing beside my eighth-grade science experiment. This moment of scientific inquiry foreshadowed a career dedicated to questioning conventional wisdom and seeking evidence-based truths in health and wellness.

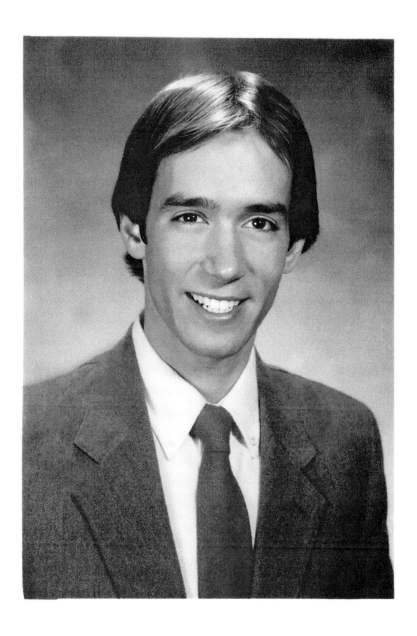

At eighteen, I was a high school graduate and ready to take on the world. My journey of discovery in health and medicine was just beginning, with many unexpected turns and revelations ahead.

Student Handbook
American Osteopathic Association

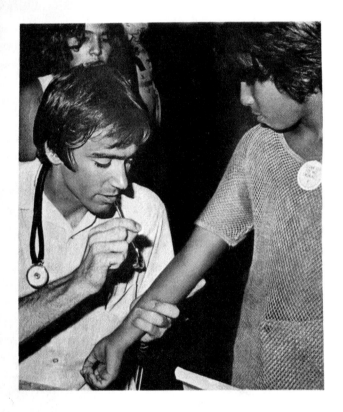

A picture of me performing a preventive screening in an inner-city Chicago clinic ended up gracing the cover of a Student Handbook for the American Osteopathic Association. This early commitment to preventive care and community health would become the cornerstone of my approach to medicine and wellness.

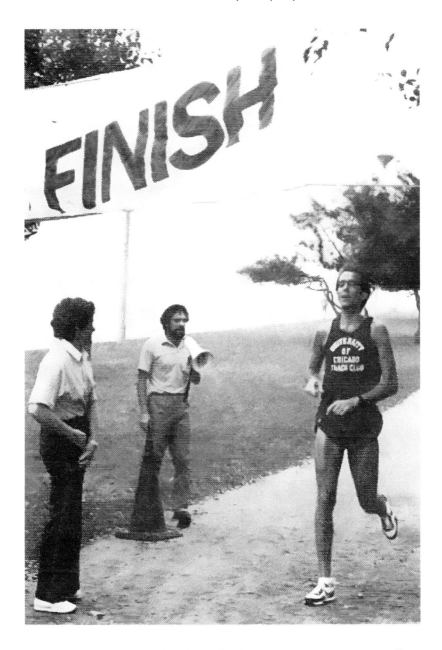

Crossing the finish line of my first and only race win: a 5K in 1980. Proudly wearing the jersey of the University of Chicago Track Club—a prestigious postgraduate athletic program I was honored to be accepted into—I shared the course with running legend Dr. George Sheehan. Ironically, the main sponsor of this race was Pfizer, a company whose approach to health I would later challenge.

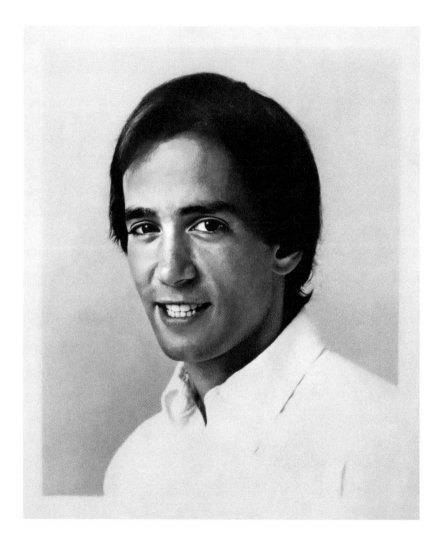

In 1982, fresh out of medical school and ready to embark on my internship. This traditional start would lead to a revolutionary journey in redefining health and wellness paradigms.

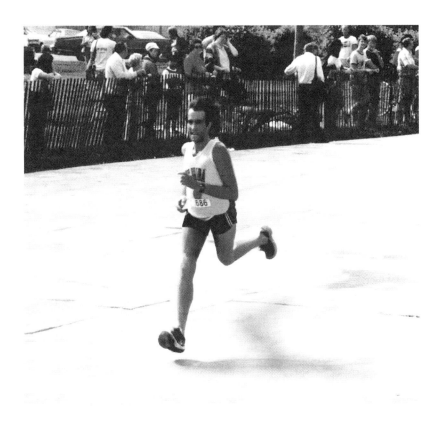

In 1985, nearing the finish line of my first and only marathon, with an impressive time of two hours and fifty minutes. This feat of endurance and dedication mirrors my relentless pursuit of optimal health and my belief in pushing the boundaries of what the human body can achieve.

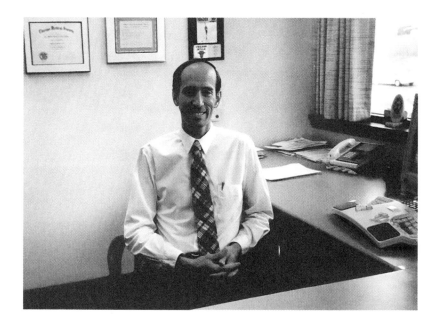

At age thirty-eight, in my suburban Chicago office, poised to input patient data into one of the first electronic medical-records systems. This moment marked a pivotal intersection of traditional medicine and emerging technology, foreshadowing the innovative approaches to health that would define my career. Unbeknownst to me, this early adoption of digital tools marked the beginning of a quest to revolutionize how we understand and approach wellness.

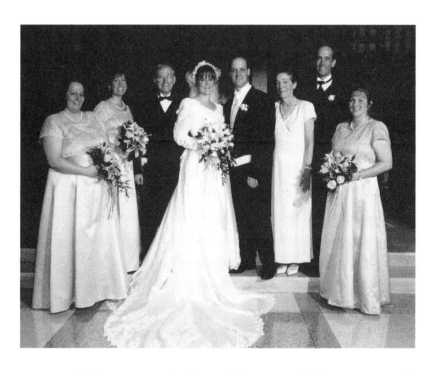

Acting as the best man at my brother's wedding, surrounded by my parents and three sisters—a support system that has been crucial in my personal and professional pursuit to revolutionize health and wellness.

In 2022, I defied conventional expectations of aging by deadlifting 405 pounds for four repetitions. This feat of strength not only highlights my personal commitment to physical excellence but also serves as a powerful demonstration of my health philosophy in action. It's a testament to how proper nutrition, targeted exercise, and a holistic approach to wellness can lead to extraordinary physical capabilities at any age, challenging our preconceptions about the limits of human performance.

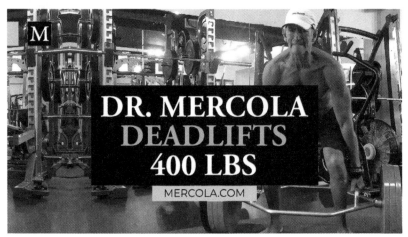

https://www.youtube.com/watch?v=gjtsc_zGPKY

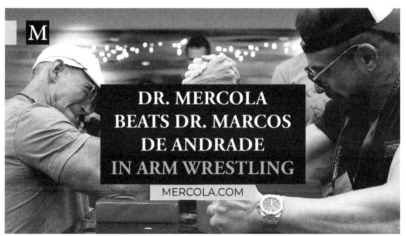

https://youtu.be/ta2iLmMwQZE

At a 2023 biohacking event in Orlando, I demonstrated the power of resistance training alongside Dr. De Andrade, an antiaging physician approximately thirty years my junior. This video shows my evolution from long-distance running to strength training over the years, reflecting my ongoing interest in health and fitness. I hope it demonstrates how staying active and adapting our routines can benefit us at any age!

Cellular Energy Is the Key to Optimal Health

Just by opening this book, you have chosen to embark on a journey of self-empowerment. This book is designed to arm you with the extensive knowledge you need to take control of your health. I have designed it to alert you to dangers we currently face—like false or underresearched claims in pharmaceutical advertising, questionable online medical information, and inept medical regulations. I want to help you cut through all that so you can make informed choices that enhance your overall well-being.

My journey begins as a young boy captivated by developments in health and technology, a passion that led me to pursue a career in medicine that's lasted over four decades and is still going strong. My mission was clear from the start: to improve not only my own health but also to enhance the health of others. This dual passion drove me to leverage the internet early on, using it as a platform to share much more about reversing illness with natural strategies than I could ever achieve alone in my medical practice in suburban Chicago at the close of the twentieth century.

For the past twenty-seven years, my website, Mercola.com, has reached hundreds of millions of people worldwide, offering a platform to question mainstream health advice. We shed light on the short-comings of a system too dependent on pharmaceuticals. These medications only manage symptoms without addressing root causes, which comes with significant costs while having minimal effect on underlying health issues. My journey through medicine and online health education has provided me with a unique outlook on the evolution of health care, as well as on the fundamental principles of biological health that remain constant.

After forty years of intensive research and countless interactions with health professionals and patients, I've gained a deep understanding of how to effectively use natural principles to prevent and reverse disease. Much of my approach builds upon the work of many unsung pioneers who came before me, whose insights have significantly shaped my thinking and teachings.

One exceptional researcher was the late Ray Peat, PhD, a biologist who developed a highly controversial set of general health principles that he codified over many decades and called Bioenergetic Medicine. Many of the concepts in this book are derived from his groundbreaking work, and I'm beyond grateful for his many contributions that have guided the evolution of my understanding of metabolic health in recent years.

Through the global COVID-19 pandemic, I advocated for a holistic approach to health as the best defense against illness. My recommendations included avoiding seed oils, engaging in regular exercise, and increasing sun exposure to boost vitamin D levels. These suggestions, rooted in my long-standing health philosophy, were violently opposed by many in the mainstream media.

Perhaps my most contentious stance was about the COVID-19 "vaccine." I warned that the rapidly developed injection was not a proven safeguard and relying on it could result in a considerable number of injuries and deaths. This stance put me at odds with mainstream medical authorities and sparked heated discussions about vaccine safety and efficacy.

This same foresight I had about COVID-19 gave me the confidence to appreciate and embrace Peat's work in Bioenergetic Medicine. I recognized its potential ahead of many others, and I'm committed to sharing these exceptional health principles with you in this book.

Among experts with a profound understanding of biological principles, there's a growing consensus that the root cause of most diseases is surprisingly straightforward: your body's inability to generate sufficient cellular energy. Cellular energy is the force that powers your body's innate drive to repair, regenerate, and recover from virtually any illness.

This is excellent news, as it gives you one goal and many tools to achieve that goal, freeing you from a dependence on expensive and ineffective medication.

The idea that cellular energy is the cornerstone of health forms what I call the "Unified Theory of Cellular Health." This theory posits that the key to preventing and curing diseases lies in optimizing the efficiency and effectiveness of cellular energy production by your mitochondria, since they produce most of your cellular energy and play a central role in metabolism. When your mitochondria function optimally, your body is well-equipped to fend off disease, repair damage, and maintain homeostasis.

The bad news is that so much of our modern lifestyle, including poor diet, environmental toxins, stress, and an overreliance on pharmaceutical interventions, often compromises your cellular energy production. These factors inevitably lead to mitochondrial dysfunction, manifesting in symptoms ranging from fatigue and minor infections to chronic and degenerative diseases.

Unlocking Cellular Health and Defending Against Modern Threats

This book is dedicated to guiding you through the complexities of recovering your cellular health. In it, you'll learn about the science of mitochondria and energy production and discover practical strategies to enhance your cellular vitality. We'll explore the impact of dietary choices, lifestyle habits, and supplements on your energy levels. Additionally, I'll provide insights into how to minimize the harmful effects of environmental toxins and other external stressors that challenge your health daily.

This book will equip you with the knowledge to make well-informed choices that increase your cellular energy, bolstering your body's innate ability to combat diseases. More than just a collection of health tips, this guide introduces a radical new perspective on health and disease, centered on restoring and optimizing your body's natural healing capabilities by enhancing your production of cellular energy.

Your ability to create abundant cellular energy is not merely a biological imperative but is the foundation on which your body constructs its defenses against aging, illness, and environmental stressors. Every heartbeat, every nerve impulse, and every breath underscore the importance of the energy that you produce and use at the cellular level. When your energy production is compromised or when the intricate balance of your energy ecosystem is disturbed, your health begins to wane—subtly at first, but then with alarming speed.

Cellular health means more than just the absence of disease. It encompasses complex interactions between genetics, lifestyle choices, and environmental factors that influence your body's energy production. This book will help you understand these interactions—how energy metabolism affects your health, and the key factors that compromise these processes, which can lead to illness.

Our exploration starts with a basic understanding of how your body generates and manages cellular energy production. We'll explore the crucial role of mitochondria, the "powerhouses" of your cells, and investigate how they produce adenosine triphosphate (ATP), the currency of your cellular energy. This foundational knowledge sets the stage for a deeper dive into the dynamics of health and disease at the cellular level.

As you navigate through this book, you'll learn how to rejuvenate your health through targeted changes in your diet, lifestyle, and supplementation practices. You'll find detailed advice on making dietary choices that provide the essential nutrients that support and enhance your mitochondrial function and cellular energy production, as well as how to eliminate mitochondrial toxins from your diet.

Moreover, you'll explore lifestyle modifications that can significantly improve your overall health, including incorporating regular physical activity, optimizing sun exposure, and eliminating harmful dietary elements. Seed and vegetable oils—canola, sunflower, and sesame, just to name a few—are the most pervasive mitochondrial toxins in your diet.

By the end of this book, you'll be equipped with the knowledge and tools necessary to make informed health decisions that enhance your ability to live a fuller, healthier, and more Joy-filled life.

The Twenty-First Century *Silent Spring*

Rachel Carson's groundbreaking work *Silent Spring* serves as a powerful reminder of how hidden environmental threats can profoundly affect our health and the world around us. Just as Carson exposed the dangers of pesticides like DDT in the 1960s, this book aims to shed light on the modern, often invisible hazards that threaten our cellular health and overall well-being.

Carson's legacy teaches us the importance of questioning the status quo, especially when it comes to substances we introduce into our environment and bodies. Her work not only sparked a revolution in environmental awareness but also showed how scientific knowledge, when clearly communicated, can drive societal change and policy reform.

Carson's work reminds us that our health is inextricably linked to the health of our environment. Just as the widespread use of pesticides had far-reaching consequences on ecosystems and human health, the modern threats we face—from endocrine-disrupting chemicals in synthetic materials to the electromagnetic fields that surround us—have equally complex and interconnected effects that lurk unseen, accumulating over time.

This book, like *Silent Spring*, seeks to connect the dots between these environmental factors and the rising tide of chronic diseases and health issues you and your family may be experiencing today. By understanding these connections, you can begin to see the bigger picture of how your daily choices and the products you use impact not just your individual health, but the health of your community and the planet.

Moreover, Carson's work underscores the importance of taking a precautionary approach to new technologies and unnatural substances. In an era of rapid technological advancement and chemical innovation, it's crucial that you critically examine the potential long-term impacts of these developments on your health and environment. This book will equip you with the knowledge to do just that—to look beyond the surface and question the hidden costs of modern conveniences.

Empowering Yourself with Informed Choices for Optimal Health and Longevity

As you embark on this exploration to uncover the secrets of optimal health and longevity, you'll find yourself navigating treacherous waters as part of the modern food landscape. It's easy to feel overwhelmed and adrift in a sea of conflicting information and hidden dangers. But amid the chaos there's a beacon of hope, a life raft that can carry you to the shores of lasting health and vitality: the power of informed choice.

In today's world, where convenience reigns supreme and the pursuit of profit often trumps well-being, the industrial food supply has become a toxic stew of chemical compounds and processed abominations masquerading as sustenance. From the deceptive allure of processed convenience foods and elegant restaurants to the empty promises of fortified cereals and breads, the average grocery store has become a minefield of hidden hazards—a labyrinth of false health claims and subsidized poisons.

You might find yourself drawn to these convenient options, seduced by the siren song of quick and easy meals, unaware of the insidious toll they take on your body and mind. As you navigate the aisles in a state of confusion, you're bombarded by labels that promise health and vitality, while the true path to wellness—the whole, unprocessed foods that nourished your ancestors for generations—remains on the periphery, unembellished by additives.

This is a testament to the pervasive influence of the industrial-food complex, a system so entrenched and interconnected that it can feel like a conspiracy against your own well-being. But the truth is there's no single puppeteer pulling the strings behind the scenes. Rather, it's a conspiracy of ignorance, a collective forgetting of the fundamental principles of health and the intrinsic value of real, whole foods.

This mass amnesia extends beyond just your food choices. It speaks to a deeper disconnect from your own spirit, the innate wisdom and resilience that lie within you. In your fear and isolation, you've become like an island unto yourself, surrounded by a vast ocean of uncertainty and misinformation.

To help you understand the gravity of the situation, let me share a powerful analogy that will forever change the way you view the hidden dangers lurking in your world. My mother grew up smoking Lucky Strikes during World War II, when the perils of smoking weren't yet widely understood. Like so many others of her generation, she picked up a cigarette, unaware of the devastating consequences that would follow. Physicians, too, were ignorant of the risks, and so the habit spread, unchecked and unquestioned.

But as time passed and knowledge grew, the truth about smoking became impossible to ignore. Those who once smoked with impunity were now faced with a choice: continue down a path of self-destruction or embrace the opportunity to change your fate. Sadly, my mom's life was cut short by emphysema, due to her choice.

In much the same way, there are pervasive, silent killers that have appeared in your environment over the last century, insidiously eroding your health and vitality by destroying the very foundation of your health: the ability of your mitochondria to generate cellular energy. Unlike smoking or recreational drugs, where the choice to partake is your own, environmental toxins are often forced upon you, infiltrating every aspect of your life without your consent.

From the plastics that surround you to the hormones and drugs you unwittingly consume in tap water, from the electromagnetic fields that bombard your body to the toxic fats that have become a staple of your diet—these silent killers are everywhere, hiding in plain sight. And yet, the odds are high that you're unaware of the devastating impact they have on your health.

Cutting Through Deception with Knowledge, Technology, and Innovation

Just as knowledge proved to be the catalyst for change in the face of smoking's dangers, so too can it empower you to take control of your health in the face of these pervasive threats to your cellular health. By understanding the nature of these silent killers and the ways in which they infiltrate your life, you can make informed, educated choices to eliminate them, reclaiming your vitality and securing a brighter, healthier future.

In just five minutes—the time it takes to smoke a single cigarette that steals eleven minutes of your life—you could instead invest in activities that not only reclaim those lost minutes but potentially add months of vibrant living to your future. By dedicating mere minutes to implementing the strategies outlined in this book, you're not just neutralizing the damage caused by mitochondrial poisons—you're actively reversing it.

It's a powerful trade-off—minutes now for months of vitality later. By choosing to invest your time this way, you're not just extending your life; you're enhancing its quality, paving the way for a future brimming with wellness and vigor. The choice is clear.

It is important to understand that there is a way forward, a route to reclaiming your health and your connection to yourself and others. And that path begins with knowledge—allowing you to make informed choices in the face of overwhelming odds. This book is a guiding light that illuminates your course to true, lasting health. With every page you turn, you're taking a step toward a life of boundless energy, radiant vitality, and the freedom to live your life with the fullest Joy possible.

By diving deep into the science of cellular energy and the root causes of disease, you can arm yourself with the knowledge you need to navigate these treacherous waters. In the pages that follow, I will give you the tools to identify and eliminate these silent killers from your life.

The Mercola Health Coach app is an innovative comprehensive digital tool created to empower your efforts to take control of your health. It offers personalized guidance, evidence-based information, and practical resources tailored to your unique health profile and goals. By integrating cutting-edge nutritional science, lifestyle recommendations, and tracking capabilities, the app serves as a virtual health companion, helping you make better, more informed decisions.

We're also building a Health Coach team consisting of health professionals from a variety of medical fields, including pharmacists, to provide personalized guidance, and we have created a handy app as an adjunct to this book.

Health-care providers in the US write over 6 billion prescriptions every year for a population of about 350 million. This staggering statistic breaks down to seventeen prescriptions per person each year. Chances are you are currently taking one or more medications yourself. By exploring alternatives and reducing your reliance on medication, you can better take control of your health.

To that end, our Mercola Health Coach has a team of trained and licensed doctors of pharmacy. They have deep knowledge and have taken a transformative leap in their careers. They have extensive experience in liberating people from their reliance on medications. These professionals now know that drugs only treat symptoms.

More often than not, this worsens health problems instead of fixing them. With this insight, they have changed their role and now aim to free people from their dependency on prescription drugs. These pioneering pharmacists are not filling bottles. They seek to help you repair and regenerate your body back to the health you deserve.

I encourage you to approach this journey with curiosity, openness, and a commitment to positive change. Your health, and indeed the health of our planet, depends on the choices you make every day. This book is your road map, and the corresponding app is your compass. Together, they will guide you toward a life filled with the health, longevity, and the Joy you deserve. You're doing so much more than reading—you're embarking on a transformative experience.

Congratulations on taking this step toward well-being, to opening your mind to the possibilities that await, and to embracing the power that lies within you to make new choices that will change your life forever. And as you do, you're not only transforming your own life—you're becoming a guide for others. By embodying the principles of true health and vitality, you'll inspire those around you to awaken to their own potential, to question the status quo, and to demand something better for themselves and their loved ones.

This is the power of knowledge. Trust in your own ability to transform your health. The rewards are immeasurable.

Let us begin.

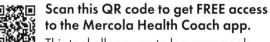 **Scan this QR code to get FREE access to the Mercola Health Coach app.** This tool allows you to log your meals, track your macronutrient ratios, and monitor your progress over time.

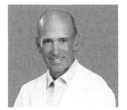

CHAPTER 1

Embrace Your Journey to Vibrant Health and Renewed Energy

Meet Kimberly, a thirty-five-year-old office manager whose story might sound familiar to you. Like many of you, she is constantly juggling her demanding job and family time while attempting to maintain a healthy lifestyle. Kimberly thought she was doing everything right. She ate low-fat foods, chose whole grains, and exercised when she could. So, when she was diagnosed with type 2 diabetes, she was utterly shocked. How could this happen to someone trying so hard to be healthy?

Let us peek into Kimberly's daily routine and uncover the hidden dangers lurking in her supposedly "healthy" choices. You might be surprised to find some of your own habits reflected in her story.

Each morning, Kimberly pours herself and her kids bowls of cereal. The boxes are plastered with health claims like "heart-healthy" and "packed with essential vitamins and minerals." What the box does not prominently announce is how much sugar and preservatives are also packed into this common breakfast option.

On days when she has more time, Kimberly opts for oatmeal, thinking it is an even healthier choice. But she does not know that most nonorganic oats are drenched in glyphosate, a harmful herbicide used to dry the oats during harvest. I have been warning people about the dangers of glyphosate for years, yet it has sneaked its way into so many of our "health" foods.

Come lunchtime, she opts for a salad with grilled chicken from a popular fast-food chain. Sounds healthy, right? Wrong. The salad is topped with dressing that is packed with inflammatory seed oils. And don't get me started on the chicken. Most commercial chickens are fed diets high in omega-6 fats from—you guessed it—more seed oils. This creates a domino effect of inflammation in your body. As for the rest of the salad, the iceberg lettuce provides minimal nutrition, and the few token vegetables are coated in preservatives.

Dinner might be a "lean" frozen meal or a stir-fry made with "heart-healthy" vegetable oil. However, the small print reveals a long list of unpronounceable ingredients and preservatives. The vegetables are mushy and overcooked, and the "lean protein" is a highly processed meat substitute that derives most of its calories from seed oils. Even the apple she has for dessert is not as innocent as it looks. It has been sprayed with 1-Methylcyclopropene, a chemical that keeps it looking fresh long past its natural lifespan.

Sound familiar? You might be nodding your head, recognizing some of your own go-to "healthy" options. Unfortunately, despite her good intentions, Kimberly's diet was rich in refined carbohydrates and hidden sugars. When Kimberly's doctor pointed this out, she switched to a low-carb diet, expecting her health to improve. To her dismay, her condition only worsened. This is where it gets interesting. Pay close attention if you have similar health issues.

The Real Culprit: Vegetable and Seed Oils

The true villain in Kimberly's diet—and yours—was not carbs or sugar. It was her excessive intake of vegetable oils and seed oils. These oils were hidden in everything she ate, from her salad dressing to her "healthy" frozen dinners. Even her attempts to cook at home often involved using these oils.

You might be wondering, "But aren't these oils supposed to be good for us?" That is what we have all been told, right? Well, hold on to your hats, because I am about to drop a truth bomb that might shake up everything you thought you knew about healthy eating.

Here is the deal: seed and vegetable oils are primarily omega-6 fats. Conventional wisdom tells us these fats are "essential" because your body cannot make them on its own. But—and this is a big but—you only need about 1,000 to 2,000 milligrams of these fats daily. Guess how much Kimberly was consuming? A whopping 60,000 milligrams every single day!

Where was it all coming from? Safflower oil, sunflower oil, corn oil, and soybean oil. These oils are everywhere in processed foods, and they are often marketed as healthy alternatives to saturated fats. Kimberly's intake of linoleic acid (LA), the main fat found in seed oils, exceeded 25 percent of her total daily calories.

To put that in perspective, before her grandmother's generation, people consumed only 1–2 percent of their calories from this type of fat. This dramatic increase—we are talking twenty times more—is a recipe for disaster. And it is not just Kimberly. If you are eating a standard American diet, chances are you are in the same boat.

How Omega-6 Overload May Be Holding You Back

Let's talk about what all this excess omega-6 is doing to your body. First up, it causes whole-body inflammation. This is important because inflammation is a significant factor in insulin resistance. When your cells become less sensitive to insulin, your body struggles to regulate blood sugar levels. Over time, this forces your pancreas to make more insulin. It eventually leads to pancreatic dysfunction and type 2 diabetes. That is what happened to Kimberly.

But that is just the beginning. These oils are changing the composition and function of your cellular membranes, which hinders your mitochondria. They cannot efficiently transport and oxidize fat, leading to fat accumulation and obesity. Think of your mitochondria as the powerhouses of your cells. When they are not working properly, your entire body suffers.

Insulin resistance is also harming your mitochondria by disrupting energy-sensing pathways in your cells. There is an enzyme called

AMP-activated protein kinase (AMPK) that acts like a metabolic master switch in your cells. When these pathways are disrupted, it can lead to obesity and fatigue. You are not just gaining weight. You are losing energy. This mitochondrial dysfunction and lower AMPK activity are messing with your appetite hormones: leptin and ghrelin. The result? Increased appetite and overeating. You are not just eating more but craving more.

And let's not forget about oxidative stress. Harmful oils lead to the formation of oxidative metabolites that can damage your cellular tissues and proteins. They also cause more of your LDL cholesterol, the "bad" kind, to oxidize, which contributes to artery-clogging plaque.

Finally, all this is causing high blood pressure, or hypertension. It is a key part of metabolic syndrome, a group of conditions that can harm your heart health, including high blood pressure, high blood sugar, excess belly fat, and abnormal cholesterol levels.

How Birth Control Might Be Clouding Your Clarity

Another piece of Kimberly's health puzzle, one that might be relevant to many of you, is birth control. Kimberly had been taking birth control pills for many years. What she did not realize, and what many women do not know, is that the pill causes weight gain in some women, especially in their abdomen. This type of fat is intricately linked to metabolic syndrome.

Birth control pills often impair your glucose metabolism as well. This leads to insulin resistance. They also harm your cholesterol by raising triglycerides and LDL ("bad") cholesterol, and lowering HDL ("good") cholesterol, which increases the risk of heart disease.

Birth control pills serve an important function in women's lives; however, if you are using or considering long-term use of oral contraceptives, get regular checkups. Your doctor should monitor your blood pressure, cholesterol, and glucose levels. It is also wise to discuss other contraceptive options with your doctor in case the pills do not turn out to be a viable option for you.

Kimberly's story is a wake-up call. It shows how our well-intentioned efforts to be healthy can backfire when we are not armed with the right information. The food industry has done a masterful job of marketing processed foods as healthy options, but as you can see, the reality is very different.

The Corporate Puppet Masters Behind Your "Healthy" Choices

Let me tell you something I have learned after decades in this field: the food and drug industries are not in the business of health. They are in the business of profit. And they have gotten incredibly savvy at manipulating us into buying their products, often at the expense of our well-being.

Take direct-to-consumer advertising, for instance. Only the United States and New Zealand allow drug companies to advertise prescription drugs directly to consumers. It is a practice that I have been railing against for years. These ads are crafted to play on your emotions, making you believe you need their latest pill to live your best life. They highlight benefits but mumble through side effects. This skews your view of the drug's safety and efficacy.

But it gets worse. These companies do not stop at advertising—they have wormed their way into the very research we rely on to make decisions about our health. It is a practice called sponsored research, and it is far more insidious than you might think.

Companies provide financial backing for studies on their products, which might sound good in theory. The more research, the better. But here is the catch: industry-funded research is often designed from the ground up to make the product look good. They might cherry-pick participants, use bad control groups, or skew data to favor their product.

Even more disturbing, if a study starts showing unfavorable results, these companies often pull the plug early. There is no law requiring all research to be published, so negative findings can be swept under the rug. It is a legal way for these companies to manipulate science, and it affects your view of their products.

The Vioxx Scandal: A Cautionary Tale

Let me share a story that perfectly illustrates the dangers of this corporate influence. Back in 1999, Merck introduced a painkiller called Vioxx. They touted it as a breakthrough, claiming it caused fewer stomach problems than other painkillers. I smelled a rat from the start. In fact, I wrote an article in my newsletter warning my readers about the cardiovascular risks of Vioxx before it even hit the market.

Turns out, I was right to be suspicious. By 2000, research was showing that Vioxx significantly increased the risk of heart attacks and strokes. A 2001 study found that patients taking Vioxx had four times the risk of heart attack compared to those taking a different painkiller. But rather than pulling the drug from the market, Merck continued to aggressively promote it, downplaying the risks and emphasizing the benefits.

In 2004, a large study showed a doubled risk of heart attack and stroke in long-term users of Vioxx. Only then did Merck withdraw the drug from the market. But, by then, the damage was done. Some estimates suggest as many as sixty thousand people may have died due to Vioxx-related cardiovascular events. That is more than the number of Americans who died in the entire Vietnam War, all because a company put profits over people's lives.

The fallout was massive. Thousands of lawsuits were filed, and Merck eventually agreed to a $4.85 billion settlement in 2007. But no amount of money can bring back the lives lost or undo the suffering caused.

Breaking the Cycle of Confusing Health Rules

You might be wondering, "But don't we have regulations to prevent this sort of thing?" We do, but here is the rub: the very agencies meant to protect us are often influenced by the industries they are supposed to regulate.

It is called the "revolving door," and it is a major problem in our regulatory system. It's common for executives from pharmaceutical or food companies to hold key positions in agencies like the FDA (Food and Drug Administration) or USDA (United States Department of Agriculture). And when government regulators leave their posts, they often end up in cushy jobs with the very industries they were previously responsible for regulating.

This blurring of lines between regulators and industry creates conflicts of interest. It is one reason why harmful products often stay on the market too long.

The Vioxx scandal, Kimberly's routine, the marketing, the biased research—they all paint a grim picture. But knowledge is power. By educating yourself, you are starting to regain control of your health. Next, we will explore how to navigate this minefield of misinformation so you can learn to make informed healthy choices for yourself and your family.

Celebrity Health Secrets You Never Knew You Needed

In today's world, celebrity endorsements wield incredible power over our health choices. These stars are not just selling products; they are selling lifestyles and dreams. When our favorite actor raves about a new supplement or a pop star swears by a certain diet, it is hard not to be swayed. I have seen many patients fall for celebrity-endorsed health fads, but they often end up in disappointment.

Social media has supercharged this effect. Influencers are the new celebrities. Their perfect lives and curated feeds have reinforced this trend. They share their opinions and all their daily routines, and it feels like they are talking directly to us. This makes their product tips more personal and trustworthy. It's like getting advice from a friend—except this friend is being paid to influence your choices.

The health sector is particularly vulnerable to this type of marketing. We all want to look and feel our best. When a physically fit, glowing influencer credits a product for their looks, it is tempting to think you are just one purchase away from the same results. But remember, what you see is often a carefully constructed illusion.

Let us talk about a prime example of celebrity endorsements gone wrong: the Kim Kardashian QuickTrim and Shape-Ups debacles. Kim and her sisters heavily promoted QuickTrim, a weight-loss supplement, claiming it was the secret to their famous figures. Millions of people rushed to buy it, hoping for similar results.

Alas, the product came under fire for deceptive marketing. Users reported no weight-loss benefits, and worse, concerns were raised about the safety of its ingredients. Consumers reported side effects ranging from cramping to kidney failure. It all ended in a lawsuit and a $5 million settlement. This was not just a case of a product not living up to the hype—it was putting people's health at risk.

The Shape-Ups story is equally troubling. Kardashian endorsed these Skechers shoes, claiming they could help you lose weight and tone muscles just by walking. But the Federal Trade Commission challenged these claims, resulting in a $40 million settlement. These cases show how easy it is for celebrity endorsements to mislead you. They can trick you into making choices that are not just ineffective but harmful.

The Self-Care Revolution You Never Knew You Needed

Now, you might be thinking, "I'm too smart to fall for celebrity endorsements." But these marketing tactics aim to bypass your rational mind and tap into your emotions. It's not about logic; it's about psychology.

Companies use advanced data mining to create ads that feel personalized. They prey on your fear of missing out (FOMO), your desire for social validation, and your craving for instant gratification. It is a powerful cocktail that can lead even the most levelheaded person to make impulsive decisions.

This is particularly dangerous when it comes to health products. We are all looking for quick fixes and miracle cures. When an ad promises rapid weight loss or instant pain relief, it is tempting to try it. But these quick-fix solutions often mask underlying health issues and can lead to long-term problems.

You Can Break Free from the Ultra-Processed Food Trap

Let's take a step back and look at how dramatically our eating habits have changed over the past half-century. Back in 1970, only about fifteen out of every one hundred Americans were considered obese. Fast-forward to today, and that number has skyrocketed to forty-two out of every one hundred. That's nearly triple!

What happened? Well, our entire food landscape transformed. In 1970, home-cooked meals were the norm, and dining out was a special treat. Today, you cannot drive down a street without passing multiple fast-food joints and convenience stores. The US now ranks among the top fifteen most obese countries globally.

This shift coincides with the rise of ultra-processed foods. These products are everywhere, from your grocery store shelves to your office vending machine. They are designed to be irresistible, with the perfect balance of salt, sugar, and fat to keep you coming back for more. But while they might satisfy your immediate cravings, they are often nutritional wastelands.

Ultra-processed foods are engineered for maximum taste and convenience, but minimal nutrition. They are typically high in calories, but low in the nutrients your body really needs. It is like filling your car with fuel that makes the engine run, but slowly damages it over time.

These foods have become so commonplace that many people do not even realize how much of their diet consists of ultra-processed items. From your breakfast cereal to your late-night snack, these foods have infiltrated every meal. They are quick, they are easy, and let's face it, they are designed to be delicious. But the cost to your health is too high.

The prevalence of these foods explains a lot about our current health crisis. They are a major contributor to the obesity epidemic—but the damage goes beyond just weight gain. Ultra-processed foods are also linked to increased risks of heart disease, diabetes, and even certain cancers. It is a stark reminder that convenience often comes at a cost.

Unmasking Health Myths and Hidden Dangers in Dietary Choices

This chapter highlighted our modern health choices and their hidden dangers. From Kimberly's so-called healthy routine to society's changing diets, corporate interests and clever marketing have warped our view of health.

The sophisticated use of behavioral psychology in advertising has made it increasingly difficult to make rational decisions. Marketers have exploited our desires for social validation, fear of missing out, and instant gratification. They have created an environment where impulsive buying of health products is now the norm.

We have seen how celebrity endorsements and influencer partnerships leverage your emotions and aspirations, often leading you astray from healthy choices—and how the food and pharmaceutical industries can prioritize their profit over your well-being.

To add to the chaos, there has been a dramatic transformation in the American diet over the past several decades. Ultra-processed foods, designed for taste and convenience, are low in nutrition. Their rise has caused a huge increase in obesity and related health issues.

As you move forward, it is crucial to approach your health choices with a critical eye. By learning the tactics that influence your choices, you can reclaim your health. Many "healthy" products are not what they seem. True health is not in a celebrity-endorsed supplement or a quick fix. It is in informed choices and a return to real, whole foods.

CHAPTER 2

The Empowering Truth About Reclaiming Your Gut Health

Imagine waking up in the middle of the night, jolted from sleep by an intense, unrelenting itch. That's exactly what happened to me on a warm summer night in 2009. I found myself battling a mysterious rash that appeared suddenly, covering my arms from shoulders to wrists. The sensation was unlike anything I had ever experienced before—a burning, insatiable itch that refused to be ignored.

As a physician, my first instinct was to reach for the usual remedies. I tried everything I could think of. I used ice packs to numb the irritation. I applied calamine lotion to soothe my skin. I used prescription steroid creams to reduce inflammation. I took oral antihistamines to calm the itching. I even tried near-infrared light therapy to boost healing. Nothing seemed to work. Each attempt at relief was met with frustration as the rash persisted, defying all conventional treatments.

Days turned into weeks, weeks into months, and still, the irritation remained. It was like trying to silence a faulty car alarm in the neighborhood. Every remedy was like pressing a different button on the key fob, hoping it would finally quiet the incessant noise. But no matter which button I pressed or how many times I tried, the alarm kept blaring, disrupting the peace and wearing down my patience.

My skin had become that stubborn car alarm, resistant to every attempt at resetting it, leaving me exhausted and desperate for silence. The constant discomfort began to take its toll, affecting my sleep, my work, and my quality of life.

It wasn't until several years later, after I had moved to Florida, that I stumbled upon a temporary remedy: aloe vera gel. The cool, soothing properties of the aloe provided blessed relief, calming my irritated skin for about an hour at a time. It wasn't a cure, but it was the first thing that had given me any respite from the constant itching.

From that moment on, aloe became my close companion. I began cultivating my own aloe plants, carefully preparing and carrying fresh aloe leaves with me wherever I went. Each day, I would slice open several thick leaves, filleting them to expose the healing gel inside. For longer trips, I'd harvest dozens of leaves, ensuring I always had a supply on hand.

But using aloe vera gel as a frequent treatment came with its own set of challenges. The gel would often leave stubborn brown stains on anything it touched—from clothing to furniture. After a few hours, the plant pieces would begin to ooze, creating a messy situation in whatever bag I carried them in. To combat this, I started double bagging the aloe. I used a thick, bright orange bag as an outer layer for puncture resistance. This orange bag became a familiar sight to my friends and staff. It was a reminder of my battle against my mysterious ailment.

How a Mysterious Rash Transformed My Medical Journey

As time went on, the rash evolved. What had started as an area of intense itching began to develop into tiny, firm nodules that resembled small mosquito bites. When I couldn't resist the urge to scratch, these nodules would transform into fibrotic, hard lumps that persisted on my arms for up to two years. The physical manifestation of the rash was now as stubborn and unyielding as the itch itself.

This was frustrating. I had a reputation as a physician who could quickly and effectively diagnose rashes. I built a career on my ability to identify and treat skin conditions. I helped countless patients find relief from their dermatological issues. But when it came to my own case, I was completely stumped. Despite my years of experience and expertise, I was unable to solve the puzzle of my own persistent rash.

But I didn't stop at self-diagnosis. I sought out expert dermatologists, hoping their unique knowledge would shed light on my condition. Even these consultations proved fruitless. The rash remained a mystery, defying classification and resisting all attempts at treatment. It was a humbling experience, to say the least, and one that forced me to confront the limitations of my own medical knowledge.

But as is often the case in life, what seemed like a curse eventually became a blessing in disguise. My struggle with this mysterious rash ignited a burning curiosity within me. I found myself driven to dig deeper, to question everything I thought I knew about health and disease. This *itch* sparked a quest for more knowledge. It led to groundbreaking insights into the complex relationship between our bodies and our environment.

I began to explore new areas of research. I peered into the human body's intricate workings and its interactions with the environment. I started to see connections that had previously eluded me and began to piece together a puzzle that was far more complex than I had ever imagined.

This journey of discovery reminded me to stay curious and question old assumptions. It taught me that, sometimes, the most valuable lessons come from our greatest challenges. As I explored gut health and its effects on our well-being, I found that my personal struggle had opened up a whole new world for me. It offered me ways to understand and treat many health issues.

Looking back, I can see how this fifteen-year battle with a mysterious rash became a turning point in my career and in my approach to medicine. It humbled me, challenged me, and ultimately led me to uncover new connections that could help millions of others. The experience was tough, but it reminded me that in health and medicine, there is always more to learn and discover.

Your Dental Fillings May Hold the Key to Recovering Your Clarity

Have you ever considered that the source of a health problem might be sitting right in your mouth? I certainly didn't. Not until a fateful night in December 1990 when I watched a riveting episode of *60*

Minutes titled "Is There Poison in Your Mouth?" This eye-opening exposé shed light on the controversy surrounding the use of mercury in dental amalgam fillings. As I sat there, eyes glued to the screen, I realized that the very fillings in my teeth could be silently wreaking havoc on my health.

Driven by this newfound awareness, I made the decision to have my mercury fillings removed. At the time, I was still practicing conventional medicine and hadn't yet transitioned into natural health. I chose a dentist who was an elder at my church, thinking I was making a safe and informed decision. Unbeknownst to me, this choice would lead to one of the biggest health challenges of my life.

Back then, I was painfully unaware of the protocols for safely removing mercury fillings. Years later, I learned about biological dentists. They use strict methods to limit mercury vapor and particles during removal. Unfortunately, this knowledge came too late to prevent the health issues I would face, but it's a crucial piece of information that I now share with everyone I can.

Here's a shocker: dental amalgam makers are the biggest users of mercury in the world! These "silver" fillings are about 50 percent mercury. In the United States alone, up to 4.2 tons of mercury each year is used for this purpose. Even more alarming, they have never been tested for safety, as required for other medical implants under US law. This is a glaring oversight that puts millions of people at risk every single day.

Let's be clear about what we're dealing with here. Mercury is not just any metal—it's a potent neurotoxin. In fact, it's ten times more toxic to neurons than lead. Mercury from dental amalgams can easily reach your brain because your mouth is so close to it. The mercury can also affect your central nervous system. It's like having a ticking time bomb in your mouth—slowly releasing poison into your system, day after day.

Dental amalgams are the biggest source of mercury exposure for most people. The World Health Organization (WHO) confirmed this in 1991. It stated that dental amalgams expose people to mercury levels that exceed safe limits for food, air, and water. Autopsy studies found dental amalgams cause 60–95 percent of mercury in human tissues. That's not just alarming, it's downright terrifying!

The effects of mercury exposure are wide-ranging and can be severe. They include everything from coughing and fever to tremors, hallucinations, memory loss, and neurocognitive disorders. Pregnant women and their newborns are particularly at risk. What makes mercury even more of a threat is that mercury vapor from dental amalgams is odorless and invisible. You could be exposed to lethal concentrations without even realizing it until it's too late.

The Dental Revolution You Never Knew You Needed

After learning about these dangers, I couldn't just sit back and do nothing. That's why I became the major funder of a nonprofit group called Consumers for Dental Choice. Their mission is vital: to ban dental amalgam. It's not just about protecting patients, it's also about safeguarding dental workers who are exposed to this hazard daily.

The leader of this organization, Charlie Brown, is a force to be reckoned with. As a former Attorney General for West Virginia, he brings a unique blend of legal expertise and strategic thinking to the table. Charlie built a global coalition that has achieved results I could only have dreamed of when we started this journey. Can you imagine my excitement when I heard about the ban on amalgam in all twenty-seven nations in the European Union? Or when I learned about individual countries in Asia, Africa, and the Caribbean following suit?

But it doesn't stop there. We've seen manufacturers shift their focus to alternative materials, recognizing the changing tide. And, perhaps most significantly, the 2017 Minamata Convention on Mercury is a worldwide treaty that has changed the global debate. The question is no longer whether we need to ban dental amalgam, but when and how to prevent any future suffering from this horrid medical mistake.

This hasn't been an easy fight. We've been up against what I can only describe as an iron triumvirate: the federal government, organized dentistry, and state regulators. It's a formidable opposition, to say the least. But Consumers for Dental Choice has been nothing short of brilliant in their approach. They've used a divide-and-conquer strategy. They combine law, science, coalition-building, and media outreach to tackle each opponent, one by one.

The results speak for themselves. Today, fewer than 6 percent of US posterior tooth fillings use mercury amalgam. That's a 73 percent drop from 2017 to 2022—the result of the first five years of the Minamata Convention phase down. In just over a decade, we've achieved global bans on mercury use in dentistry. It's a victory that still amazes me when I think about it.

Though this is great news for people who need fillings in the future, what about those of us who already have mercury fillings? There are over 100 million of us in the United States alone, and every year about 100 million new mercury fillings are placed. If you're one of these people, listen closely: the way these fillings are removed matters enormously.

I learned this the hard way. When I had my amalgam fillings removed, I didn't know I needed to find a dentist trained in safe removal techniques. Improper removal can release more mercury into your system, causing a cascade of harm. That's why I urge you, if you're considering having your amalgams removed, to take the time to find a qualified dentist. Charlie Brown's group, Consumers for Dental Choice, is a great resource. Their website, toxicteeth.org, has a link at the top of the page to locate dentists who are trained in the safe removal of mercury fillings.

I wish I had known about this resource earlier, which is why I'm sharing it with you now. I believe it's crucial information for anyone with amalgam fillings. Remember, when it comes to your health, especially when dealing with a potent neurotoxin like mercury, it's always better to be safe than sorry. Take the time to find the right dentist and resolve to pay more for their care if necessary. Think of it as an investment in your health. Your future self will thank you for it.

Uncover the Hidden Environmental Factors Clouding Your Health Goals

Now, let me share a personal experience that might have contributed to my health issues. A few months before my mysterious rash appeared, I took a trip to India with key members of my company and my girlfriend at the time. One day, we stopped at a small, unassuming restaurant. The open-air setup buzzed with locals, and the air was thick with the aroma of spices and sizzling food. Unfortunately, despite assurances of the food's safety, most of the people in our group soon became ill as a result of parasites derived from the local cuisine.

After my rash erupted, it occurred to me that these parasites might have played a role in its development. I underwent tests and tried many herbal and homeopathic remedies to eradicate them. Unfortunately, these efforts brought no relief to my condition. Much later I learned that although the parasites I encountered in India might not have been the culprit, the country's poor air and water quality might have had a hand in my condition. You see, India has a massive mercury pollution problem. India is the world's second-largest source of mercury pollution—mainly from coal burning.

It is now my firm belief that my time in India, coupled with the removal of my mercury fillings, created a perfect storm. The excessive mercury exposure, both from within and without, caused kidney damage. This then made me more susceptible to the ill effects of oxalates, which was the next piece of the puzzle. I'll get to that in a moment.

It's a reminder that our health can be affected by unexpected factors, from our dental fillings to the food we eat, to the air we breathe, and the water we drink. It stresses the need to be aware of these hidden dangers so we can protect our health in a toxic world.

Empowering Steps to Unlock Your Body's Balance

Let's talk about an often-overlooked powerhouse in your body: your skin. It's not just a wrapper for your insides—it's your largest organ, covering about twenty-two square feet! Your skin is a multitasker.

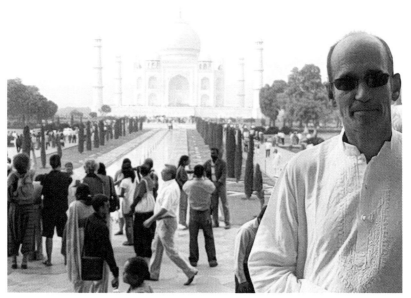

At the majestic Taj Mahal during my business trip to India, where we met with our partners at Organic India.

It shields you from bacteria and UV rays, it regulates your internal health and makes vitamin D, and it must also rid the body of toxins. That's one of its most crucial jobs.

Your skin is like a built-in detox system, sweating out waste products, excess salts, and even heavy metals. It's your body's way of cleaning house from the inside out. This natural process is amazing when you think about it—your body is constantly working to keep you healthy, even when you are not aware of it.

When I was dealing with my mystery rash, I thought I'd give my skin's detox abilities a boost. I turned to infrared saunas, using them three times a week. The idea was simple: raise my body temperature, sweat more, and hopefully flush out whatever was causing the rash. It seemed logical, right?

Well, it turns out that while saunas can be great for overall health, they weren't the silver bullet for my rash. Despite my regular use, the irritation persisted. But I didn't give up on saunas. Even though they didn't solve my specific problem, I noticed other benefits. I felt better, more relaxed, and it became a part of my routine that I looked forward to.

This experience taught me an important lesson. Sometimes, a treatment might not solve your main problem, but it can still be beneficial in other ways. It's about looking at your health holistically, not just focusing on one symptom or issue.

Relief at Last: Unveiling the Hidden Cause of My Rash and a Life-Changing Solution

Eventually, I diagnosed my rash as oxalate dermatitis. This condition has never been previously described. Oxalates are organic compounds in many foods. Your body also makes them by metabolizing molecules like vitamin C. Normally, excess oxalates are removed by your body in your urine. However, high oxalate levels can lead to a buildup of these compounds in various tissues, including the skin.

The permanent kidney damage I sustained—a result of excessive mercury exposure from improper amalgam filling removal and mercury-polluted air in India—compromised my body's ability to process oxalates. This oxalate buildup would have been prevented had I had healthy kidneys.

Your skin is not just a protective barrier. Like your kidneys, your skin excretes wastes and toxins, including excess oxalates. This happens if your body's main waste routes are overwhelmed. This is where the mechanism of oxalate dermatitis begins.

Shortly before I wrote this book, I was finally able to identify the best solution for my intense itch. It is well known that mineral citrates like magnesium, potassium, and calcium citrate bind to oxalates. These citrates are even used in the prevention of calcium oxalate kidney stones.

Sally Norton, a famous health researcher, has focused her work in this area (oxalates) and mentioned to me that a topical mixture of these minerals would be effective in the treatment of an oxalate rash. I found that glycerin could suspend these powders, so I crafted a homemade "lotion" that I could easily apply to my skin. Applying this suspension stopped the itch almost instantaneously and reduced the rash by 80 percent. It was the best remedy I had ever encountered in my fifteen-year battle with this rash!

The treatment worked so well that I could clearly see that my individual hair follicles were inflamed. This wasn't the random, diffuse redness of a mosquito bite but a precise pattern of tiny, swollen dots marking every follicle. Once I realized this, the method of how the oxalates caused the rash suddenly occurred to me. My body was trying to rid itself of excess oxalates through sweat!

This is why it migrated the oxalates to my skin. This process allowed the oxalates to congregate in my hair follicles and sweat glands. Sweating is one route for oxalate excretion and our kidneys are another. Normally, the kidneys are responsible for most of the oxalate removal. Due to the kidney damage I had sustained, my skin excretion played a much larger role in removing oxalates than it normally would have. In short, the oxalate load exceeded my body's ability to remove the oxalates without uncomfortable symptoms.

I then realized that medicine indeed had a name for my rash. Although none of the many dermatologists I visited were able to diagnose it correctly, the name is prurigo nodularis (PN). Deconstructing the Latin phrase *prurigo nodularis* reveals its meaning. It is a literal description of the condition's main symptoms. *Prurigo* translates to "itching" in English, while *nodularis* refers to the presence of nodules or small lumps. Thus, the term in its most basic interpretation signifies "itchy nodules."

I had previously considered that diagnosis but discounted it because of the range in size of the lesions. The key was having a solution for the itch that addressed the cause by removing the oxalates. I could then see that the source was the hair follicles themselves.

If the oxalates were not removed, the skin damage would continue to worsen. This damage wouldn't be limited to just the hair follicles; it would also affect the surrounding skin. In fact, the affected area could extend to ten or even twenty times the size of a single hair follicle, causing significant collateral damage. The clinical definition of the rash now fit. Especially the relentless itching, which caused an itch-scratch cycle that worsened the condition. The sleep impairment that led to anxiety and depression was also spot-on.

I believe I have now correctly identified why most people develop this condition. I also believe the more accurate term for this rash is not prurigo nodularis but oxalate dermatitis. This evolution of PN has never been described in the medical literature, so I plan to write a paper on this.

Although my proposal is speculative, it aligns with our understanding of similar processes in the body. If correct, and I believe it is, this new information would help many people avoid the needless pain and suffering I endured for so many years.

Understanding the Role of Oxalates

Here are the basics: When your oxalate load exceeds your body's ability to eliminate it, the oxalate builds up in the skin. As the oxalate concentration increases, the tissues become supersaturated, and the oxalates begin to crystallize. Oxalate crystals in the skin trigger an inflammatory response similar to other irritants, such as uric acid and calcium oxalate kidney stones. You could even consider this problem a type of skin "stone."

When present, these crystals set off a chain reaction in your body. First, pro-inflammatory cytokines are released, followed by the activation of immune cells. Cytokines are small proteins released by cells that act as signaling molecules to regulate immune responses, inflammation, and cell communication.

This then leads to increased blood flow to the affected area. These reactions are your body's standard defense mechanisms against foreign or irritating substances. In this case, oxalate crystals act as the irritant, prompting this typical inflammatory cascade associated with dermatitis—such as redness, swelling, and intense itching.

The itching sensation could be particularly severe for several reasons. Firstly, the crystals themselves can act as a physical irritant to nerve endings in your skin. Secondly, the inflammatory mediators released during the immune response are known to stimulate nerve fibers, causing the itchy sensation.

The intense itching then leads to scratching, which damages the skin. The result is a vicious cycle of irritation, inflammation, and itching/scratching that is commonly noted in many chronic skin conditions.

Here's the good news: When citrates like magnesium, potassium, and/or calcium citrate are applied to the hair follicle, they bind to the oxalates and help remove them from the follicle. As a result, the inflammatory cytokines decrease, and the itching stops.

This process can also be likened to gout, in which excessive uric acid crystallizes in the joint synovial fluid, causing inflammation. Oxalates are also an acid. Specifically, they are two carbon dioxides joined together to form dicarboxylic acid. So, a similar topical strategy could likely provide relief for gout symptoms as well.

Description of Prurigo Nodularis

Prurigo nodularis (PN) is a chronic skin condition. It causes nodules to become intensely itchy and can greatly affect a patient's life. The main symptom of PN is severe itching. It's often described as a burning or stinging sensation. The itching can be constant or intermittent and usually worsens at night. This itching causes an itch-scratch cycle that worsens the condition—disrupting sleep and eventually causing anxiety and depression.

Physically, PN manifests as firm, round-to-oval nodules ranging from 0.5 to 3 cm in diameter. These nodules are usually on the extensor surfaces of the limbs, trunk, and, occasionally, the face. They are symmetrically distributed. Their appearance can range from skin-toned to reddish or dark in color. They often look darker than the surrounding skin. The nodules have a characteristic hard, sometimes waxy or scaly texture.

Frequent scratching often damages the skin around and between the bumps. The skin becomes thicker, with more pronounced lines, and darker in color. In chronic cases, scarring may occur, leading to permanent skin changes. The areas between nodules may appear dry, and patients might even develop nail changes due to chronic scratching.

The appearance of PN can vary depending on the stage of the disease. It may start as small, red, itchy bumps. In chronic stages, it has larger, defined nodules with other skin changes. Some nodules may coalesce to form larger plaques.

Unlike many other pruritic conditions, in PN, the itch often precedes the development of skin lesions. The nodules are well-defined and elevated, with a symmetrical distribution. This helps to distinguish PN from other nodular skin conditions. Chronic scratching leaves marks, harms the skin, and deteriorates the quality of life for the affected person.

Embrace the Secret to Cellular Renewal You Never Knew Existed

As I reflect on my journey, I'm struck by how far I've come. My path in health and medicine has been anything but conventional. It all started in Chicago in 1968 with a computer programming class. From there, I went on to establish my solo medical practice in Schaumburg, Illinois. I've always had a passion for both technology and health, and this unique combination led me to launch Mercola.com in 1997.

Over the next twenty years, my website grew to become the most-visited natural-health site. It has allowed me to help hundreds of millions of people worldwide. But it was my personal health crisis—this fifteen-year battle with the mysterious, persistent rash—that truly transformed my approach to medicine and healing.

This experience sparked a journey of discovery for me. I explored the links between cellular energy, gut health, and well-being. It pushed me to question everything I thought I knew about health and disease, and to look for answers in places I'd never considered before.

With this new knowledge, I set out to restore my cellular energy. I wanted to revive my mitochondria and help my beneficial bacteria thrive again. I sought to heal and recover. I used new methods to nourish my cells, support my gut, and detox my body.

Slowly but surely, as my cellular energy levels began to rise, I saw a transformation. The rash that had been with me for so long began to fade—the inflammation subsiding as my body's natural balance was restored. My gut bacteria and revived mitochondria gradually eliminated the oxalates in my skin.

This newfound wisdom has freed me from a fifteen-year health challenge. It has also sparked a sense of awe and potential I never knew existed. It's as if every cell in my body is humming with renewed energy and vitality. I find myself smiling more, laughing more easily, and embracing each day with a sense of wonder and appreciation.

But my quest hasn't stopped there. This new theory of health has also offered me insights into many other health issues. This breakthrough has opened a new chapter in my career. I now have new tools and understanding to help others avoid physical pain and suffering in their lives.

This approach isn't just for my rare condition. It can help solve almost any health challenge you face. Granted, it's not a cure-all and may not work for everyone. But I believe it can help with, if not fix, 90–95 percent of the health issues out there.

What sets this theory apart is that it tackles the foundational causes of health problems in a way that no other system has before. It's about the links between cellular energy, gut health, and well-being. It's about recognizing that our bodies are complex systems. True healing often requires addressing multiple factors at once.

As I stand here today, looking back on this transformative experience, I'm filled with a sense of gratitude and Joy. The trek from confusion to healing has taught me the power of perseverance. It showed me that I need to trust my instincts. And it revealed to me how deeply our bodies and minds are connected.

And now I'm eager to share this journey with you, to guide you through the fascinating world of cellular energy and mitochondrial function. I believe that, by understanding the root causes of your health issues, you too can heal. You can reclaim your vitality. And you can live the vibrant, energetic life you were meant to live.

CHAPTER 3

Unlock Your Body's Potential for Vibrant Health and Endless Energy

The root cause of most health problems isn't what your doctors have been telling you. It's not just about diet, exercise, or your genes. The real culprit: a decrease in cellular energy. The tiny powerhouses in your cells aren't working as they should and are wreaking havoc on your health. This lack of cellular energy harms your microbiome, which is a complex ecosystem of trillions of microorganisms in your gut.

You might be thinking, "What's the big deal about some bacteria in my intestines?" Your microbiome is vital to your health. It affects your metabolism, immune system, and brain function. When your gut bacteria are out of balance (a condition called dysbiosis), a host of health problems can crop up, like obesity, diabetes, and mental disorders.

The good news is that by restoring your microbiome and your cellular energy, you can start to address these health challenges head-on. It's like giving your body the fuel it needs to fight back against disease. I've seen it work firsthand.

In addition to curing my persistent rash, my sleep needs changed dramatically. I used to need seven to eight hours to feel rested. Now

I'm thriving on just five hours a night. I wake up naturally, feeling refreshed and ready to tackle the day. But here's the most surprising part—I grew taller. Yes, you heard that right. Using a precise laser measurement device, I documented an increase in height of nearly one inch. Now, I'm not saying everyone will grow taller, but it just goes to show how profound the effects of improved cellular energy can be.

The importance of cellular energy cannot be overstated. It underpins every single process in your body—from your heart beating to your brain thinking—it all requires energy at the cellular level. The high rates of illness we're seeing in this country are a clear indicator that nearly everyone in the US has radically decreased cellular energy production.

Insulin Resistance: Simple Steps to Reclaim Your Metabolic Power

Now, let's talk about a key player in this whole energy crisis: insulin resistance. This is a metabolic process gone haywire, and it's intimately linked to the health of your microbiome. When your gut bacteria are out of balance, it leads to insulin resistance. Addressing insulin resistance is crucial to restoring optimal cellular energy.

So, what exactly does insulin do? If you think of your body as a booming metropolis, insulin is the traffic controller that makes sure everything runs smoothly. In a healthy system, insulin efficiently directs glucose, the fuel that powers your cellular citizens. But when insulin resistance sets in, this smooth operation starts to falter.

It's like a gradual breakdown in communication between the traffic controller and the vehicles it directs. The controller's signals become muffled, forcing it to shout louder and more frequently just to keep traffic moving. In your body, this translates to higher levels of insulin production as it struggles to manage blood glucose effectively.

This seemingly small glitch in the system can cascade into a city-wide crisis. As insulin loses its effectiveness, glucose builds up in your blood. It can't reach its intended destinations.

Meanwhile, your pancreas works overtime, pumping out more and more insulin in a desperate attempt to clear the roads. The importance of recognizing insulin resistance early cannot be overstated. It's like having an early-warning system for your metabolic health. Long before signs of trouble appear, insulin resistance is at work. It silently disrupts your body's balance. These warning signs include high fasting glucose and changes in body composition.

What makes insulin resistance such a critical marker is its role as a precursor to many metabolic disturbances. It's the canary in the coal mine, often preceding type 2 diabetes, obesity, heart disease, dementia, and cancer. By the time these serious conditions show, insulin resistance has likely been present for decades, quietly setting the stage for metabolic chaos.

Interestingly, you can have insulin resistance even if you're at a normal weight or even underweight. This is why relying solely on traditional markers like body mass index (BMI) or even fasting glucose can be misleading.

The Connection Between Mitochondria, Insulin Resistance, and Disease

Mitochondria rely on proper insulin signaling to efficiently convert nutrients into energy. When insulin resistance takes hold, it disrupts this delicate process, leading to a decline in your mitochondrial energy production, which is at the core of almost every health problem we experience.

Here are a few of the many medical conditions affected by poor mitochondrial health: sarcopenia, innate immunity deficiencies, obesity, sepsis, kidney dysfunction, diabetes, osteoporosis, poor oral health, glaucoma, neurodegeneration, cognitive dysfunction, inflammation, Alzheimer's, depression, heart disease, heart failure, metabolic dysfunction, metabolic associated fatty liver disease (MAFLD), preeclampsia, nonalcoholic steatohepatitis (NASH), liver disease, bone diseases, skin aging, poor lung function, seizures, spinal muscular atrophy, skeletal muscle atrophy, COVID-19, inflammatory bowel disease (IBD), reperfusion injury, adrenal dysfunction, rheumatoid arthritis, multiple sclerosis (MS), and polycystic ovary disease.

Tired of Guessing about Your Health? Your Path to Clarity Starts with HOMA-IR

Fortunately, we have a powerful tool to measure insulin resistance: the HOMA-IR test. Developed in 1985, this test combines fasting glucose and insulin levels to give us a clear picture of how well your body responds to insulin. It's a reliable and practical test for insulin resistance and prediabetes.

What sets the HOMA-IR apart is its accessibility and reliability. Unlike complex, invasive procedures, this test needs only a blood draw. This makes it convenient for patients and practical for use in clinics. The HOMA-IR gives a clear measure of insulin resistance. It helps people and doctors spot metabolic issues early and track improvements over time. The HOMA-IR formula is as follows:

HOMA-IR = (Fasting Glucose x Fasting Insulin) / 405, where

- Fasting glucose is measured in mg/dL

- Fasting insulin is measured in μIU/mL (microinternational units per milliliter), and

- 405 is a constant that normalizes the values

If you're using mmol/L for glucose instead of mg/dL, the formula changes slightly:

HOMA-IR = (Fasting Glucose x Fasting Insulin) / 22.5, where

- Fasting glucose is measured in mmol/L

- Fasting insulin is measured in μIU/mL, and

- 22.5 is the normalizing factor for this unit of measurement

So, what's considered a healthy HOMA-IR score? Anything below 1.0. If you're above that, you're considered insulin resistant. The higher your values, the greater your insulin resistance. Insulin resistance often exists long before obvious signs of trouble, silently disrupting your body's balance and setting the stage for serious conditions later.

Incidentally, my personal HOMA-IR score is 0.2, which is incredibly low. In fact, it's the lowest Dr. Cate Shanahan, who introduced me to HOMA-IR, has ever seen. The reason for this is that my body became more efficient at burning fuel, due to the increased availability of glucose. I consumed extra carbohydrates, which gave my cells energy. They could function better, which improved my metabolic health.

Now, I know some of you might be worried about the idea of increasing your carbohydrate intake. After all, we've been told for years that carbs are the enemy, right? Well, I'm here to tell you that it's not that simple. Yes, insulin resistance and fat gain are valid concerns, but they can be effectively managed with the right approach. However, don't use my experience as a reason to drastically increase your carbohydrate intake. What worked for me may not work for everyone, especially if your microbiome is not in a healthy state. Eating more carbs without fixing your gut can harm your health. It may cause insulin resistance and fat gain.

I recommend healing your microbiome first. I explain how to do this in chapter 12. This will boost your carbohydrate metabolism, allowing you to safely add more diverse kinds of carbs to your diet without ill effects.

The Shocking Truth about Insulin Resistance: It Affects 99 Percent of Americans

According to Dr. Shanahan's analysis of the most recent CDC National Health and Nutritional Examination Survey (NHANES) data, over 99 percent of the US population has insulin resistance. Let that sink in for a moment. Nearly everyone in this country is facing this metabolic challenge. But addressing insulin resistance early can help.

You can do this with lifestyle changes or with targeted interventions that can halt or even reverse the progression to serious metabolic disorders. It's like doing routine maintenance on your city's infrastructure. It prevents small issues from becoming major crises.

A major consideration when battling insulin resistance is what's going on in the microbiome in your gut. Imagine your gut lining as a brick wall, with insulin acting as the mortar holding it together. When insulin resistance sets in, that mortar starts to crumble, weakening the entire structure. This breakdown causes "leaky gut," a condition where substances that should stay in your gut slip into your bloodstream. This can cause many health issues.

But that's not all. The high blood sugar that comes with insulin resistance becomes a feast for pathogenic bacteria. It's like leaving a buffet for unwanted guests. They'll multiply, tipping your gut's ecosystem out of balance. This shift can harm your health, causing inflammation and immune issues.

The connection between insulin resistance and gut health is a two-way street. As your gut health declines, it can further exacerbate insulin resistance, creating a vicious cycle. Breaking this cycle is crucial for restoring both gut health and metabolic balance.

Embrace Your Inner Microbiome: A Guide to Nurturing Your Gut Allies

Let's take a journey back in time—way back to the origins of life on Earth. The Oparin-Haldane theory suggests that life began in an oxygen-free environment. This would mean that the earliest life forms had no defenses against oxygen because they never needed them. Instead, they were adapted to living in a completely different atmosphere than what we have today.

This might seem like ancient history, but it's incredibly relevant to your health today. Some of these ancient, oxygen-intolerant bacteria are still with us, playing a crucial role in your gut health. They're like living fossils, carrying on their ancient ways in the oxygen-free environment of your colon.

Knowing this history helps you see why gut health is so vital. It's not just about feeding yourself. It's about nurturing an ancient ecosystem that's been part of human biology for millions of years.

Your colon is home to a staggering 95 percent of your body's microbes, and they're not all created equal. On one side, you have the oxygen-intolerant bacteria, ancient warriors that thrive in the absence of oxygen. These are the good guys, the ones we want to nurture. They're like the wise elders of your gut, carrying out crucial functions that keep you healthy.

On the other side, you have the oxygen-tolerant bacteria, more adaptable fellows that can switch between aerobic and anaerobic respiration. While they have their place, an overgrowth of these bacteria

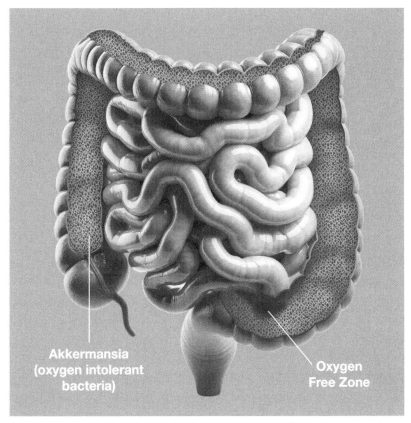

Akkermansia *is a keystone gut microbe that requires an oxygen-free environment to thrive.*

will cause you trouble. It's like having too many party crashers at a carefully planned event—they disrupt the delicate balance and will lead to all sorts of problems.

A balance between these two types of bacteria is required for good health. When oxygen-intolerant bacteria dominate, they create a gut-healthy environment that boosts your well-being. But when oxygen-tolerant bacteria take over, it leads to inflammation, digestive issues, and even systemic health problems.

The following illustration paints a vivid picture of this microbial battle. On one side, we see the beneficial bacteria, their numbers dwindling as oxygen seeps in. On the other, the oxygen-tolerant bacteria, their cell membranes studded with harmful endotoxin, are ready to unleash their evil payload.

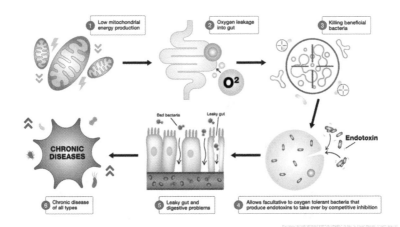

As mitochondrial energy production is reduced, oxygen levels in your gut rise, causing beneficial bacteria to perish while oxygen-tolerant, endotoxin-producing bacteria thrive. The endotoxins released can trigger widespread inflammation, impacting overall health.

Two Alternative Medicine Practices That Might Unwittingly Disrupt Microbial Balance

Understanding that the interior of your large intestine should be free of oxygen makes it clear that two alternative medicine practices might need reconsideration. Specifically, rectal insufflation of ozone and the use of hyperbaric oxygen, both of which increase oxygen levels in your intestine and could potentially diminish the population of these beneficial oxygen-intolerant bacteria.

Although there are currently no studies directly evaluating the impact of these interventions on the microbiome, I am planning research later in 2024, which will include pre- and post-intervention microbiome analysis to validate this concern.

Regrettably, I once not only personally used these therapies but also recommended them to others, unaware of the microbiome concerns I just shared. The insights I have since gathered make it evident that such therapies should be used with caution. While conditions may exist that warrant interventions like hyperbaric therapy, they should be followed by rigorous efforts to restore and maintain a healthy population of oxygen-intolerant bacteria.

Your Gut's Hidden Heroes Will Help You Reclaim Your Vitality

Your colon maintains a controlled oxygen gradient that is crucial for the growth of oxygen-intolerant bacteria. It's like having different climate zones within your gut, each supporting specific types of bacterial life. This gradient isn't static; it requires a constant supply of cellular energy to maintain.

If that energy supply falters, oxygen can seep in, killing off your beneficial bacteria. As beneficial bacteria dwindle in numbers, more harmful, oxygen-tolerant species gain ground. This imbalance then sets the stage for a range of other health issues.

Maintaining this oxygen gradient is one of the most important, yet often overlooked, aspects of gut health. It's not just about what you eat, but about creating the right environment for your beneficial bacteria to thrive. This is where the importance of cellular energy production comes into play. Without it, the entire system can collapse.

And what do we have to thank for maintaining this system? Some of the hardest-working cells in your body: colonocytes and goblet cells. Colonocytes line your colon walls, performing many vital functions. They're like the bouncers at an exclusive club, deciding what gets in and what stays out. They also play a crucial role in maintaining that all-important oxygen gradient.

Goblet cells, on the other hand, are the maintenance crew. They secrete a mucus that acts as a protective coating, shielding your gut lining from harmful substances and pathogens. Colonocytes and goblet cells form a strong defense for your gut.

The health of these cells is directly linked to your overall gut health and, by extension, your general well-being. When they work well, they help build a strong gut barrier, absorb nutrients, and balance the microbiome. But when compromised, it can lead to many digestive and systemic health issues.

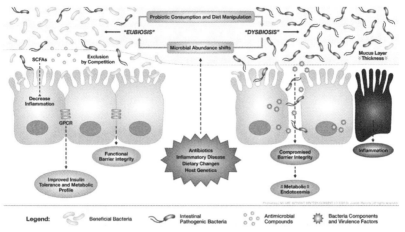

This illustration depicts the delicate balance of gut microbiota and its impact on health. On the left, "Eubiosis" shows a healthy gut environment with beneficial bacteria, strong barrier integrity, and positive metabolic outcomes. On the right, "Dysbiosis" demonstrates how factors like antibiotics and an inappropriate diet can disrupt this balance, leading to inflammation and compromised gut health. Probiotic consumption and diet can cause dramatic shifts in microbial abundance, influencing everything from mucus-layer thickness to insulin tolerance and metabolic profile.

Embrace Your Inner Ecosystem and Finally Gain Control of Your Weight

Here's another fact you might not know: the bacteria in your gut have a direct impact on your weight. It's not just about calories in and calories out, as we've been led to believe for years. The loss of some beneficial bacteria, especially one called *Akkermansia*, is a major cause of today's diabetes and obesity epidemics. These bacteria are vital for more than digestion. They help produce hormones, especially GLP-1, which regulate appetite and blood sugar.

You might be wondering, "How can tiny bacteria have such a big impact on my weight?" Well, it's all about that delicate balance in your gut. When you lose the beneficial strains, it's like removing the gatekeepers of your metabolism. Without them, your body struggles to regulate blood sugar, control appetite, and maintain a healthy weight. It's a domino effect that can lead to a host of metabolic issues.

Unfortunately, the conventional medical approaches to losing weight often ignore this crucial factor. They're too busy prescribing pills and pushing fad diets instead of looking at the root cause of weight gain. Nurturing your gut bacteria will help you control your weight and health. No pill or crash diet can do that.

Now, let's talk more about a condition I mentioned earlier that's the source of so many health problems: leaky gut. As I said before, when your gut is working properly, it lets in the good stuff (nutrients) and keeps out the bad (toxins and undigested food particles). But when the balance is disrupted and those foreign invaders slip into your bloodstream, it isn't just a digestive issue, it's a full-body crisis.

When these unwanted particles enter your bloodstream, your immune system goes into overdrive. It's like setting off the alarm system in your body, triggering inflammation and a cascade of immune responses. This constant state of alert can lead to a whole host of health issues.

We're talking about skin issues, like eczema and psoriasis, and autoimmune diseases, like rheumatoid arthritis and lupus. Even conditions like chronic fatigue syndrome and fibromyalgia have been linked to leaky gut. The conventional medical approach often fails to make these connections. It treats each symptom in isolation, instead of addressing the root cause. But by focusing on healing your gut, you can resolve a wide range of seemingly unrelated health issues.

The Modern Assault on Your Gut: Unmasking the Culprits

Let's face it: our modern lifestyle is at war with your gut health. Processed foods, which make up a large part of the standard American diet, are like poison to your beneficial gut bacteria. They're full of vegetable oils, additives, and artificial ingredients. Your body can't handle them.

But it's not just about food. Excessive alcohol consumption is another major player in gut disruption. It's a biological poison that not only kills off beneficial bacteria, but also damages the lining of your gut. And let's not forget about stress—in our fast-paced world, chronic stress has become the norm, and it is wreaking havoc on our digestive systems.

Some medications, especially antibiotics and NSAIDs, can also disrupt your gut flora. And for those with digestive diseases like

Crohn's or ulcerative colitis, the challenge is even greater. It's a perfect storm of factors that leads to widespread gut dysfunction and the health issues that come with it.

The Alcohol Deception: It's Worse Than You Think

Alcohol isn't just bad for your liver, it's a full-body assault, and your gut is on the front lines. When you drink alcohol, your body treats it like the poison it is, prioritizing its metabolism more than anything else. It's converted into acetaldehyde, a highly toxic substance that wreaks havoc on your cells.

But the damage doesn't stop there. Alcohol directly inhibits your mitochondria, which we know are the tiny powerhouses in your cells that produce energy. Mitochondrial dysfunction reduces energy production, which affects every system in your body.

And let's not forget about insulin resistance. Alcohol is a major cause of this condition. It leads to type 2 diabetes and other metabolic disorders. It's a direct path to liver disease, gut inflammation, and systemic health issues. The occasional drink might seem harmless, but the cumulative effects can be devastating.

Love Your Gut and Unlock the Rapid Wellness You Never Thought Was Possible

It's vital to understand the link between energy production, gut oxygen levels, and your microbiome to reclaim your health. It's all interconnected, like a delicate ecosystem. When one part is out of balance, it affects everything else.

Your mitochondria produce the energy your body needs to function. This energy is used, in part, to maintain the proper oxygen gradient in your gut. This gradient, in turn, allows your beneficial bacteria to thrive. These bacteria then produce compounds that support your mitochondria. It's a beautiful, symbiotic cycle when it's working properly.

Your microbiome plays a crucial role in how you process food, produce vitamins, and even how you feel emotionally. That's right, there's a strong gut-brain connection that the mainstream medical community is just beginning to recognize.

Your gut microbiome even plays a crucial role in regulating your immune system. Those tiny bacteria in your intestines are key players in keeping your immune responses in check. Think of your microbiome as a training ground for your immune system. It teaches your immune cells the difference between friend and foe. Without this education, your immune system might misfire, causing autoimmune diseases. By nurturing your microbiome, you can support a balanced, effective immune system naturally.

Let's talk about something your doctor probably hasn't told you about—short-chain fatty acids (SCFAs). These fats are produced by beneficial gut bacteria when they ferment fiber. And let me tell you, they're true health heroes.

SCFAs protect against colon cancer. New research suggests they may prevent other cancers, too. How? They influence the cell-growth process, helping to keep cell division in check. In cancer, cell growth goes haywire. SCFAs help put the brakes on this process.

SCFAs also act as signaling molecules, communicating with various systems in your body. They help regulate your immune system, reduce inflammation, and even influence your metabolism. It's like having a team of tiny health managers working 24/7 to keep you in top shape.

These incredible compounds are also crucial for maintaining your gut barrier. In fact, SCFAs supply a whopping 70 percent of the energy needed by the cells that line your colon. Your gut cells prefer these bacterial by-products over glucose!

These SCFAs are broken down through a process called beta oxidation. This process uses a lot of oxygen, which helps maintain the low-oxygen environment that your beneficial bacteria need to thrive. It's yet another beautiful example of the symbiotic relationship between your gut bacteria and the internal environment of your colon. A fiber-rich diet boosts your body's SCFA production. You're not just feeding yourself but also your gut's guardians.

GLP-1: The Gut Hormone That Could Change Your Life

Another factor we need to recognize is a hormone you might not have heard of but that plays a crucial role in your health: GLP-1. This hormone is made by special cells called L cells that reside in your colon. It's a game-changer for regulating your blood sugar and appetite.

GLP-1 is a master controller. It tells your body when to release insulin, slows stomach emptying, and signals your brain that you're full. It's nature's own appetite suppressant and blood sugar regulator, all rolled into one.

The production of GLP-1 is stimulated by certain gut bacteria, particularly *Akkermansia*. This is one of the reasons why maintaining a healthy gut microbiome is so crucial for metabolic health. Nurturing your gut health, especially the *Akkermansia*, with a healthy diet boosts your body's GLP-1. This helps control blood sugar and manage weight naturally.

The pharmaceutical industry has caught on to the power of GLP-1 and created synthetic versions of it, like Wegovy and Ozempic, for weight loss and diabetes treatment. But why rely on an expensive drug when you can support your body's natural production?

Additionally, let's talk about something the pharmaceutical industry doesn't want you to know. GLP-1 agonist drugs like Wegovy and Ozempic are hailed as miracle cures for obesity and type 2 diabetes, but they are not the harmless solutions they're made out to be. Sure, they mimic the action of GLP-1, but they don't address the root cause of why your body isn't producing enough GLP-1 in the first place.

And let's not forget about the potential long-term consequences. We're talking about creating a dependency on a synthetic hormone. Once your body starts relying on this external source, it could reduce its own natural production even further.

What's more, these drugs can run you up to $20,000 a year! That's highway robbery for something your body should be producing naturally, if given the right conditions. It's another example of how the drug industry profits from our metabolic dysfunction, rather than helps us fix it.

Your Gut Bacteria Hold the Secret to Improving Your Foggy Mind and Tired Body

Something else you need to consider is a by-product of oxygen-tolerant bacteria in your gut: endotoxin, which we will cover in more detail in the next chapter. This waste product is a major cause of death in the US, although you won't hear about it from mainstream medicine. When pathogenic bacteria take over your gut, the resulting endotoxin overload can lead to septic shock.

Septic shock conservatively kills an estimated three hundred thousand Americans each year. That's more than breast cancer and prostate cancer combined. Endotoxin overload is also a common trigger for heart failure, which affects one in four Americans. It's linked to cancer and neurodegenerative diseases like Alzheimer's and Parkinson's too. The scary part is this process is happening silently, without most people—including many doctors—even realizing it.

This might sound like a lot to process, but we're just scratching the surface when it comes to understanding how your gut microbiome affects your overall health. New research links gut bacteria to diseases you never thought would be related. Take cystic fibrosis, for example. It's the most common genetic disease among Caucasians, and there's growing evidence linking it to gut microbiome imbalances.

Recent studies have also found that people with glaucoma have lower levels of butyrate-producing bacteria in their gut. Butyrate is one of those amazing SCFAs we talked about earlier. This connection opens exciting new possibilities for prevention and treatment of this condition.

I'd bet my bottom dollar that, as research progresses, we'll find that most diseases are related to the microbiome in some way. It's a paradigm shift in how we think about health and disease, and it is high time the medical establishment caught up.

The bottom line is, if you want to achieve true health, you've got to address the causal factors. Popping pills to mask symptoms isn't going to cut it. You need to dig deep and tackle the root causes of your health issues. And often, that root cause can be traced back to your gut.

This is especially true when it comes to managing leaky gut. You need to identify what's causing the damage in the first place. Is it a poor diet? Chronic stress? Environmental toxins? All the above? Once you find the culprits, you can make the appropriate changes that will heal your gut and improve your health.

Now, I'm not saying making these changes is going to be easy. It requires a broad approach that considers the complex links among your diet, cellular energy, and your microbiome, rather than just your waistline. But let me tell you, it's worth it.

You realize that food affects more than your waistline. It impacts your energy and gut bacteria. Chronic stress isn't just making you feel frazzled. It's disrupting your gut barrier and harming your immune system. You start to see that environmental toxins are not just "out there." They're harming your cellular energy and disrupting your microbiome.

This holistic view empowers you to make informed decisions about your health. It's not about following a one-size-fits-all diet or popping the latest "miracle" supplement. It's about understanding your body as a complex, interconnected system and giving it what it needs to thrive.

Throughout this chapter, we've peeled back the layers of deception surrounding your health. We've seen how the pharma industry pushes drugs like GLP-1 agonists. We've explored the effects of leaky gut and the deadly consequences of endotoxin overload. We've found new links between the microbiome and diseases like cystic fibrosis and glaucoma. And to battle all this and more, we've stressed a holistic approach that considers diet, cellular energy, and the microbiome.

The central theme is clear: your gut health is the foundation of your overall health. The conventional medical approach often misses this. It focuses on treating symptoms, not root causes. You can control your health in ways no drug can. Nurture your gut microbiome, boost your cellular energy, and avoid toxins.

Armed with this knowledge, you're now equipped to make better informed decisions about your health. We must move beyond the Band-Aid solutions of conventional medicine. We need a holistic approach that addresses the root causes of health issues. Your body has an incredible capacity to heal when given the right tools. A focus on gut health, cellular energy, and toxin protection will bring true, lasting health and vitality.

Transform Fatigue into Vitality by Tackling the "Four E's" of Cellular Health Risks

In the ongoing battle to protect your health, four formidable adversaries, which I refer to as the four E's, stand out.

These cellular foes can harm your well-being. They are:

- Excess essential fats like linoleic acid (LA)

- Estrogen and estrogen-like chemicals from plastics (xeno-estrogens)

- Electromagnetic fields (EMFs) from electronic devices

- Endotoxins from oxygen-tolerant gut bacteria

An excess of any of these four E's can disrupt energy production. Excess essential fats, particularly those found in vegetable or seed oils, slip right past your cell's defenses like a Trojan horse. Once inside your body, they infiltrate your mitochondria, disrupting the flow of energy and causing the cell to stall.

Estrogen is a hormone that can become a turncoat when there's too much of it. Estrogen-like chemicals leach from plastics and microplastics into your food and water. These chemicals are also pervasive in personal care products, and even the air you breathe. Excess estrogen, like a double agent, infiltrates your cells and disrupts your mitochondria's ability to generate energy. This throws your entire system into disarray.

EMFs are a silent, insidious poison. They penetrate your cells and disrupt the balance of ions and electrons. This balance is crucial for your mitochondria to work properly. All these toxins have the same result: a buildup of the fourth E. Endotoxin, a by-product of bacteria, attacks your cells like a battering ram against a castle's gates. It overwhelms your cells' defenses so that toxins and damaging free radicals pour into your cells.

The relentless assault of the four E's makes energy production erratic and unreliable. Your mitochondria, once the proud power plants of the cellular city, struggle to generate even a fraction of the energy they once produced. Your cells, robbed of their life force, begin to die. This sets the stage for health problems that can ravage your body.

Excess essential fats, estrogen, endotoxin, and EMFs harm your cells and hurt their integrity and function. By knowing this, you can find ways to protect and support these vital building blocks of life. Avoiding these four E's as much as possible supports your mitochondria, which is essential if you are to recover your health.

The First E: Essential Fats Found in Vegetable and Seed Oils

At the time of the American Civil War (1861–1865) virtually none of these mitochondrial poisons existed. But toxic influences would soon become all too common. As the nation emerged from the ashes of war, a new threat arose. This threat came in a seemingly innocent form. It was a golden elixir that promised to revolutionize cooking—cooking oil extracted from seeds and, later, from vegetables such as canola, a member of the brassica family.

Soybean oil currently leads the market in terms of production and usage, followed by palm, canola, sunflower, and corn oils. Peanut, safflower, sesame, grapeseed, cottonseed, rice bran, and flaxseed oils are also common. Once processed, these fats cause oxidative stress and mitochondrial damage. These oils are hard to avoid as they are pervasive in the food supply, from processed foods to restaurant meals.

The 1870s saw the start of oil production, especially cottonseed oil. New technologies made it possible to extract and refine oils on a massive scale. To understand the full impact of consuming these oils, you must first dive into the very building blocks of your cells: the fats that make up your cell membranes.

These fats come in two types—saturated and unsaturated. They determine the health and function of every cell in your body. Saturated fats have been in the human diet for millennia. Despite what you have been told about their impact on heart disease, their stable structure and resistance to oxidation make them ideal for your body. But with the rise of vegetable and seed oils, a new type of fat began to dominate: polyunsaturated fats, or PUFAs.

These PUFAs, which include omega-3 and omega-6 fats, are essential in small amounts. You must consume them because your body can't make them. But as with most things, there is a point at which too much becomes dangerous. Seed oils, when consumed, incorporate into your cell membranes. They displace the stable saturated fats that have served us well for so long. This process can take years, but sets the stage for destroying your health and underlies nearly every modern chronic disease.

Why Most Studies That Evaluate the Effects of Consuming Seed Oils Are Misleading

The link between seed oils and chronic diseases is full of contradictions. Some studies suggest that vegetable and seed oils may protect against diseases like diabetes. Others say they could worsen the condition. These conflicting results can be frustrating. But you must understand the factors behind them to see the bigger picture.

One crucial aspect to consider is the design of the studies themselves. Differences in the studied populations can greatly affect the results. These factors include age, gender, and health. For instance, a study on young, healthy people might yield different results than one on older adults with health issues. This can lead to contradictory

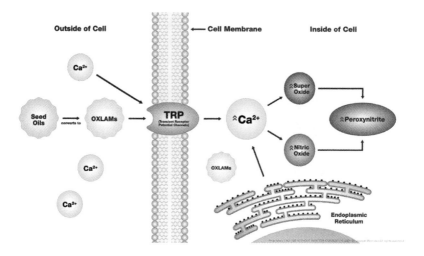

Cellular Calcium Signaling and Oxidative Stress. This diagram illustrates the complex interplay between seed oils, calcium ions, and cellular oxidative processes. On the left, seed oils convert to OXLAMs (oxidized linoleic acid metabolites) outside the cell. These, along with extracellular calcium ions (Ca2+), activate TRP (transient receptor potential) channels in the cell membrane. Inside the cell, this activation leads to increased calcium levels, triggering the production of superoxide and nitric oxide. These reactive species combine to form peroxynitrite, a potent oxidant. The endoplasmic reticulum, shown at the bottom right, plays a crucial role in calcium storage and release. This cascade of events shows how dietary components like seed oils can influence cellular signaling and potentially contribute to oxidative stress, highlighting the intricate connections between nutrition and cellular health.

findings if the results are not interpreted appropriately. This makes it hard to draw clear conclusions about the health effects of seed oils.

Additionally, the context in which seed oils are consumed plays a crucial role in the findings. Your diet, including other nutrients, can alter how your body metabolizes seed oils, which changes their effects on your health. A diet high in antioxidants might reduce some of the harm of seed oils. But a diet low in protective nutrients could worsen their effects.

Some antioxidants, vitamins, and minerals can mitigate harm from seed oils. Vitamin E, for instance, protects seed oils from oxidation. It thus reduces its harmful effects, including metabolic issues and fatty liver. Carnosine, another key player, absorbs reactive oxygen species (ROS) and advanced lipoxidation end products (ALEs) in order to spare your mitochondria, DNA, and proteins.

However, it's not all good news. The way you prepare your food can affect the risks of eating vegetable and seed oils. High-temperature cooking can increase the tendency of PUFAs to oxidize rapidly and create harmful compounds. Frying or roasting foods at high temperatures using seed oils creates toxic substances. This may negate any benefits and actually add new health risks.

Another factor contributing to the contradictory findings is the duration of the studies. Some focus on immediate effects, while others examine long-term outcomes. This difference in timeframes leads to opposing conclusions. It complicates the data's interpretation. Short-term studies might show minimal harm or some benefits. Long-term studies typically reveal the damage from prolonged seed oil use.

The primary fat in vegetable and seed oils is linoleic acid (LA). These highly industrially processed oils are likely the single most damaging metabolic poison in your diet. LA is essential for your health in small amounts. But as we've said, too much causes chronic disease, mainly due to its harmful effect on your cellular energy production.

Seed oils don't just pass through your body. Instead, they undergo metabolic transformations that have profound implications. These changes lead to a loss of the energy so crucial for maintaining your well-being. Low energy makes your cells less efficient and more prone to damage and illnesses such as heart disease and metabolic syndromes like diabetes and obesity. Energy depletion also promotes the growth of oxygen-tolerant bacteria, kicking off its own negative health cascade.

But Isn't Linoleic Acid an Essential Fat?

As an omega-6, LA is considered an "essential" fat that your body can't function without. While this is true, the idea that you are at risk of deficiency is based on flawed studies from the late 1920s and early 1930s. We will discuss the flaws of these studies later. The truth is LA is so common in food, it's nearly impossible to become deficient in it unless you stop eating altogether.

This raises a critical question: How did we go from thinking of LA as "essential" to consuming such wildly excessive amounts? The answer is a mix of historical, scientific, and industrial factors. They have shaped our view of and use of these fats over the past century.

Historical evidence suggests that human diets originally provided fewer than two grams and possibly as low as half a gram of LA per day. This stark contrast to our current consumption shows a big shift in our diets. Recent findings suggest that most people consume over 20 grams of LA daily, in large part thanks to the vegetable and seed oils used in cooking and processed food. That's about 6 percent of their total daily calories. However, our real biological need is closer to just half a gram.

This huge gap between our needs and our consumption is a recipe for metabolic disaster. LA has a half-life of 600 to 680 days (about two years). It will stay embedded in your cells for years, gradually leaking out and converting into toxic metabolites that poison your mitochondria. Its prolonged presence in your body means that, even if you cut back today, it could take several years to clear out the harmful LA and its by-products that are currently in your body.

Researchers have indeed noted a disturbing trend in the concentration of LA in human fat tissue. Between 1959 and 2008, the concentration of LA in fat tissue increased by a staggering 136 percent! This increase is highly correlated with the rise in dietary LA intake over the same period.

The pervasiveness of seed oils in the modern food supply makes it challenging to avoid them entirely. They're marketed as healthier alternatives to traditional cooking fats. The widespread use of these oils, combined with decades of bad dietary advice, has led most people to consume far more LA than their bodies can handle.

To make informed diet choices, you must know LA's history and its current level of consumption. LA is essential in small amounts. But the evidence shows our intake is far too high. It's beyond what's healthy. Reducing your seed oil intake will help you shift to a healthier diet. To do this, you need to recognize the gap between your needs and your consumption.

The Eye-Opening Truth You Never Knew About Seed Oils

The sharp rise in seed oil use has coincided with a rise in health issues. One of the most striking examples is the surge in heart disease rates. Arthur Firstenberg's book *The Invisible Rainbow* explores old data on heart disease rates from the early 1900s. He notes that, back then, heart disease was rare in the US. It was the twenty-fifth most common cause of death. This is a stark contrast to today's figures, where heart disease has climbed to the top of the list, currently holding the number one spot.

To put this into perspective, according to the CDC (Center for Disease Control), heart disease was responsible for about 695,000 deaths in the United States in 2021 alone. This accounts for roughly one in every five deaths, making it the leading cause of death for both men and women across most racial and ethnic groups. This shift is staggering. It should wake up anyone worried about their heart health.

But heart disease isn't the only health concern that has seen a dramatic uptick alongside the increased consumption of seed oils. Cancer mortality rates have also surged alarmingly. In 1811, the cancer mortality rate was about one in 118 individuals. Fast forward to 2010, and that rate had skyrocketed to a shocking one in three. The American Cancer Society's *Cancer Facts & Figures 2023* report predicted about 609,820 cancer deaths in the United States in 2023.

These statistics prove the widespread nature of metabolic disorders in the US population, and people often have many metabolic disorders at once. Let's break down the current situation:

Insulin resistance, the precursor to many metabolic disorders, has reached epidemic proportions. As I covered in chapter 3, by analyzing the 2015–2018 NHANES (National Health and Nutritional Examination Survey) supplemental tables, Dr. Shanahan found that over 99 percent of the US population is insulin resistant. This enormous number shows how common this metabolic dysfunction is, and it affects nearly every aspect of your health.

Prediabetes, a condition that puts you at considerable risk for developing type 2 diabetes, is also rampant. According to the CDC, as of 2020, approximately 96 million American adults—more than one in three—have prediabetes. What's even more alarming is that of those with prediabetes, more than 80 percent don't know they have it. This silent epidemic is laying the groundwork for a future surge in diabetes cases if left unchecked.

Speaking of diabetes, the CDC reports that 37.3 million Americans—about 11.3 percent of the population—have type 2 diabetes. Of these, approximately 28.7 million people have been diagnosed, while 8.5 million remain undiagnosed. This means millions of Americans are unaware they have a deadly condition.

Obesity, another condition intricately linked to metabolic dysfunction, has also reached unprecedented levels. The CDC reports that for 2017–2020, the prevalence of obesity in adults was 41.9 percent. Even more alarming, the prevalence of severe obesity was 9.2 percent.

Hypertension, or high blood pressure, is another condition that has seen a dramatic increase. According to the CDC, nearly half of adults in the United States (47 percent, or 116 million) have hypertension. This "silent killer" can cause severe heart problems if untreated.

Studies have also linked high intake of vegetable oils and seed oils to neuroinflammation and poor brain development. The link is particularly troubling considering the rapidly rising rates of neurodegenerative diseases and cognitive disorders.

The Impact of Seed Oils on Body Fat and Obesity

It's important to recognize the significant role that seed oils play in body-fat accumulation and obesity. This goes far beyond the simplistic notion of counting calories. The influence of seed oils extends to the very core of your metabolic processes and the way your body manages fat storage.

Seed oils act like master sculptors, shaping the way your body creates and stores fat cells. This process unfolds in several critical steps. It starts with their activating specific transcription factors that set the stage for the early phases of fat-cell growth. These transcription factors are like blueprints. They guide fat buildup in these cells.

But seed oil's influence doesn't stop there. They can also impact insulin sensitivity and glucose levels, which are critical factors in fat storage and distribution. While insulin promotes glucose uptake and lipid synthesis in fat cells, excessive intake of seed oils, particularly those high in omega-6 fats, contribute to insulin resistance. This disruption can lead to abnormal fat storage and increased body fat.

Seed oil's impact on your waistline is more than new fat cells. It's also about where these cells settle and their effects on your health. Research shows that diets high in seed oils tend to increase visceral fat. That's the kind that wraps around your vital organs like an unwelcome embrace. This type of fat is a key player in the development of metabolic syndrome, diabetes, and heart disease. Visceral fat also contributes to insulin resistance and worsens inflammation.

Understanding how seed oils affect your body's fat storage is key for anyone wanting to lose weight and improve their health. It shows the need to go beyond calorie counts. Instead, you need to focus on the types of fats in your diet.

Seed Oil's Complex Role in Cancer Dynamics

One of the most concerning implications of high LA consumption is its role as a primary driver of cancer. The link between LA, its by-products, and cancer is complex. It involves key processes that can greatly affect your health.

At the heart of this issue are metabolic breakdown products called oxidative linoleic acid metabolites (OXLAMs). These toxic compounds, like 4-hydroxynonenal (4-HNE), seriously damage your DNA and disrupt your body's normal functions. Faulty cellular processes can cause malignant transformations, which can lead to cancer.

But the story doesn't end there. OXLAMs create loads of reactive oxygen species (ROS) that lead to genetic mutations and maladaptive behaviors in cells that are typical of cancer progression.

ROS has been shown to act in ways that enhance the invasive capabilities of cancer cells. They can change proteins that help cells stick and move. This makes cancer cells more mobile, allowing them to invade nearby tissues and even spread to distant organs. It's like giving these malignant cells a superpowered ability to spread and wreak havoc throughout your body.

To lower your cancer risk, reduce your intake of seed oils. This is especially true for cancers linked to inflammation and oxidative stress. By opting for healthier saturated fats, you can boost your health. And you may also help your body fight this much-feared disease.

The Second E: Estrogens—Many of Which Come from Plastics

Hormonal balance is key to human health. It links our physical and emotional well-being. Excess estrogen disrupts this balance and causes a condition called estrogen dominance. This wreaks havoc on your body. The sources of this estrogen overload are many and often hidden. They include birth control pills, estrogen replacement therapy, and thousands of estrogenic compounds in plastics, pesticides, personal care products, and even clothing.

Synthetic pharmaceutical estrogens were introduced in the 1930s and became more common just before World War II. Diethylstilbestrol (DES) is a notable synthetic estrogen that was sold as a miracle drug in the treatment of many conditions, including pregnancy complications and menopausal symptoms. However, the enthusiasm for these synthetic hormones was short-lived. In the 1970s, researchers made a chilling discovery: DES was linked to a rare vaginal cancer in the daughters of women who took the drug during pregnancy.

Estrogen, when in balance, plays essential roles in your body. It's known for its involvement in energy production and coordination of reproductive health. It also provides mitochondrial support for your cardiac and skeletal muscles. But here's the catch: estrogen's primary benefits occur only when it's not present in excessive amounts. When estrogen levels spiral out of control, the very systems it's meant to support begin to break down.

The effects of estrogen toxicity are far-reaching and can manifest through many symptoms. Hormonal imbalances are often the first sign, but they're just the tip of the iceberg. Excess estrogen increases your risk of certain cancers, particularly breast and uterine cancer. It also negatively affects your mood. Weight gain becomes a persistent struggle, often resistant to diet and exercise, and the insulin resistance it causes leads to diabetes in many.

But the list doesn't end there. Excessive estrogen is a factor in fibroids, irregular periods, and endometriosis. It also causes adenomyosis, which affects one in five women, but few know of it. As if this weren't enough, excess estrogen may worsen endotoxin toxicity. This can happen through several pathways, compounding the damage to your body.

At the cellular level, the impact of excess estrogen is equally concerning. Your estrogen receptors are often overactivated by the endocrine-disrupting chemicals (EDCs) in most plastics. This significantly affects calcium regulation and mitochondrial function.

Research has shown that estrogen raises calcium levels inside many cell types. These include endometrial cancer cells, platelets, and mammalian cells. And this effect is not gradual. It's rapid and potent. It causes a big spike in calcium inside your cells within seconds of estrogen exposure.

The link between estrogen and autoimmune diseases is another crucial part of this complex puzzle. Autoimmune disorders disproportionately affect women. As many as four in five people with these conditions are female. This stark gap isn't a coincidence. It's due to women's higher estrogen levels. Between twenty-four and fifty million Americans have an autoimmune disease, which occurs when the immune system mistakenly attacks the body's own tissues.

Higher estrogen levels in women may also increase their risk of leaky gut. This triggers immune responses throughout the body, which helps explain why women are more affected by autoimmune diseases.

Estrogen enters your body in ways you might never have imagined. Your body is constantly bombarded by an invisible army of chemical invaders known as xenoestrogens. These synthetic compounds, mostly a result of microplastic exposure, mimic the effects of estrogen. They come from a mix of sources: plastic containers, pesticides, industrial chemicals, and canned-food linings.

This pervasive exposure creates a baseline of excess estrogen activity in your body, a tide that's constantly rising. Now, imagine adding more fuel to this raging hormonal fire with estrogen replacement therapy. It's like trying to navigate a ship through storm-tossed seas while deliberately adding more water to the ocean. Your endocrine system is already burdened by xenoestrogens in the environment. Any additional influx of estrogen could tip it into chaos.

For this reason, you must be extremely cautious about any estrogen therapy. I strongly recommend avoiding it. A dose that seems therapeutic might, in our xenoestrogen-saturated world, push you into estrogen dominance. This will worsen the very symptoms you're trying to fix. It might even cause serious health problems. In this chemical maze, be cautious with even the most "natural" or "bioidentical" hormones.

It's imperative to understand that estrogen is everywhere. It's not just about avoiding obvious sources of synthetic estrogens. It's also about recognizing the hidden sources that surround you every day, and these estrogen-mimicking compounds are everywhere.

This realization can be overwhelming, but it's also empowering. With this knowledge, you can take concrete steps to reduce your exposure. Start by examining the products you use daily. Look for personal care items free from parabens and other estrogenic compounds. Use glass or stainless-steel containers, not plastic ones, for storing and heating food. Choose organic produce whenever possible to avoid pesticide residues, as they too can have estrogenic properties.

Your body is resilient. It can regain balance if you support it. Reduce your exposure to excess estrogen and support your body's natural detox processes. In this estrogen-filled world, stay alert but don't be afraid. Every small step you take to reduce your exposure is a victory. It will support your body's natural balance. Your health is in your hands. With the right knowledge and choices, you can thrive despite living in a toxin-riddled world.

The Pervasive Scourge of Endocrine-Disrupting Chemicals

Your body faces a constant barrage of chemical invaders known as xenoestrogens. These synthetic compounds mimic estrogen in your body. This exposure creates a baseline of excess estrogenic activity in your body. It's a rising tide, threatening to overwhelm your natural hormonal balance.

The impact of xenoestrogens on your health cannot be overstated. They disrupt your hormonal balance, which can cause reproductive problems and metabolic disorders. It's especially alarming that xenoestrogens can affect you at extremely low doses. Sometimes, these doses are even lower than the levels of your body's natural hormones.

Let's dive deeper into the world of EDCs. EDCs include many substances. Among the most notorious are phthalates and PFAS, or "forever chemicals." These chemicals are everywhere. They are in your food packaging, plastic products of all kinds, and personal care products. They're also in countless items made by industrial processes.

The widespread presence of EDCs in our environment is nothing short of alarming. They're in the products you use every day, often without your knowledge. From the moment you wake up and brush your teeth with toothpaste in a plastic tube, to when you sit on your vinyl office chair, to the moment you lay your head on a pillow treated with flame retardants, you're in constant contact with these hormone-disrupting chemicals. It's a sobering truth, and it shows the need for awareness.

Bisphenols: The Tough Guys of the Plastics World

Among EDCs, bisphenols are notorious. Bisphenol-A (BPA) is probably the one you've heard of the most. This compound is the tough guy of the plastics world. It makes water bottles shatter-resistant and prevents food cans from rusting. But its ubiquity comes at a steep price to your health. BPA has been linked to many health issues, including hormone-related cancers, reproductive problems, and metabolic disorders.

What's particularly insidious about bisphenols is their ability to mimic estrogen in your body. They can bind to estrogen receptors and trigger responses that your body would normally reserve for its own hormones. This can cause hormonal chaos. Your endocrine system receives mixed signals and struggles to stay balanced. The effects can be particularly destructive during critical development periods, like fetal growth or puberty.

In response to public concern, many manufacturers have started producing "BPA-free" products. However, this label is radically misleading. Just because a product is BPA-free doesn't mean it's free from other bisphenols—and these alternatives are just as toxic as BPA.

These BPA alternatives often have similar chemical structures, so they have similar hormonal effects in your body. In some cases, they may even be more potent or harder for your body to metabolize than BPA. This means you should be cautious about alternatives without long-term safety data. It's not enough to avoid one known toxin if it's simply replaced with another that could be just as harmful or worse.

Phthalates: The Flexible Foe in Your Environment

While bisphenols are the tough guys, phthalates are the chameleons of the plastic world. These compounds are known for their ability to make plastics flexible and pliable. They let vinyl flooring bend without breaking and make shower curtains drape elegantly. But beneath this versatility lies a darker truth about their impact on your health.

Phthalates aren't just passive contaminants. They are potent endocrine disruptors. They activate the same estrogen receptors as natural estrogen and change how your endocrine glands make hormones. They also disrupt hormone transport, metabolism, and excretion. And they are doing all this at trace levels, meaning even small exposures can have significant impacts on your health.

Most alarmingly, these chemicals compete with your natural hormones, throwing your entire hormonal balance into disarray. Additionally, they have a signaling power sometimes thousands of times more powerful than regular hormones.

The ubiquity of phthalates in modern life is staggering. They're found in a wide array of products beyond just plastics. Personal care products, like shampoos and lotions, often contain phthalates. They help fragrances in perfumes last longer. They're in the coatings of pharmaceutical pills and nutritional supplements. They're even found in the ink used on receipts and the glues holding your shoes together. This widespread use means you are constantly exposed to phthalates.

The health impacts of phthalate exposure are broad and concerning. These compounds are linked to reproductive issues. In men, they reduce sperm count and motility, as well as raise the risk of testicular cancer and sexual problems. In women, they raise the risk of endometriosis and polycystic ovary syndrome (PCOS) and contribute to fertility issues and pregnancy complications.

They've also been tied to developmental problems in children, including altered brain development and a higher risk of attention deficit disorders. Some studies link phthalate exposure to a higher cancer risk. This is especially true for hormone-sensitive cancers, like breast and prostate cancer.

Embrace a Brighter Tomorrow by Understanding and Reducing Your Plastic Exposure

Consider this: detectable levels of BPA have been found in 96 percent of urine samples from a representative sample of the US population. This isn't just a statistic; it's a wake-up call. It means that virtually every person in the United States is carrying around this harmful chemical in their body.

Thyroid impairment is another significant concern when it comes to EDCs. Your thyroid gland plays an instrumental role in regulating metabolism, growth, and development. EDCs interfere with thyroid hormone production, transport, and action in your body. This disruption causes issues ranging from subtle changes in energy and weight to serious conditions like hypothyroidism or thyroid cancer. The thyroid is vital for early development. When EDCs disrupt your thyroid during pregnancy or early childhood, it can have severe, lasting effects.

Perhaps surprisingly, EDCs have also been associated with respiratory issues. Some of these chemicals, especially phthalates, are linked to a higher risk of asthma and allergies. The exact mechanisms aren't fully understood, but EDCs change immune responses and make the respiratory system more reactive to allergens and irritants. This is yet another example of how these chemicals have effects far beyond their primary endocrine-disrupting actions.

The cancer risk associated with EDCs is also a growing area of concern. As with phthalates, this is especially true for hormone-sensitive cancers, like breast, prostate, and testicular cancer. Some EDCs damage DNA directly, while others promote cancer cell growth or disrupt natural tumor suppression. Moreover, many cancers have a long latency period, so the full impact of your current EDC exposure may not be clear for decades.

Liver damage is another potential consequence of EDC exposure that is often overlooked. Your liver plays a crucial role in metabolizing and detoxifying chemicals in your body, including EDCs. Chronic exposure to these chemicals overwhelms your liver. It may cause inflammation, fatty liver disease, and even liver cancer. This is especially alarming as your liver is vital for good health and has a limited ability to regenerate itself.

Finally, the neurologic damage associated with EDCs is a growing area of research and concern. These chemicals have been linked to a range of neurodevelopmental and neurodegenerative conditions. Certain EDCs, when exposed to fetuses in the womb, harm children's minds and behavior. This includes causing attention deficit and autism spectrum disorders. In adults, EDC exposure may also increase the risk of Alzheimer's and Parkinson's. The brain's chemical balance is delicate, making it especially vulnerable to EDCs.

Let's put this into perspective with some numbers that will make your head spin. In 1950, global plastic production was a mere 1.5 million tons. Fast forward to 2023, and that number has skyrocketed to an overwhelming 400 million tons. But hold on to your hats because the projections for the future are even more alarming! By 2060, plastic production could reach a mind-boggling 1.2 billion tons. That's not just growth; it's an explosion.

Now, you might be thinking, "Surely we're recycling most of this plastic, right?" Wrong. By 2015, approximately 6.3 billion tons of plastic waste had been generated globally. Here's the kicker: only 9 percent of this waste was recycled. A staggering 79 percent ended up in landfills or the natural environment. In many respects, we're turning our planet into a giant garbage dump.

The oceans, often called the lungs of our planet, bear the brunt of this pollution. An estimated 8 million tons of plastic enter the oceans every year. Let that sink in for a moment. Eight million tons. Every. Single. Year. And if we continue along this path, projections suggest that by 2050, there could be more plastic, by weight, than fish in the ocean. It's a future that is hard to imagine, and even harder to accept.

But here's where the story takes an even darker turn. When you discard a plastic bottle or a shopping bag, its journey has only just begun. Over time, exposed to sunlight, wind, and water, these larger plastic items slowly fragment into smaller and smaller pieces. But they don't disappear. They become microplastics and then nanoplastics. These fragments are so tiny that they're invisible to the naked eye.

This transformation isn't a quick process. It can take up to five hundred years for many plastic items to degrade into these microscopic particles. Think about that. The plastic straw you used once and tossed away could still be breaking down when your great-great-great-grandchildren are walking this earth. And during all this time, the plastic doesn't remain inert. It becomes a pervasive source of toxicity in our environment.

These microplastics are insidious invaders in our ecosystems. Fish and other marine life ingest them, mistaking them for food. Plants absorb them through their roots. They find their way into the soil where our crops grow. And inevitably, microplastics end up on your plate and in your body. In fact, you're inhaling them with every breath, ingesting them through your food, and even absorbing them through your skin.

The extent of microplastic infiltration in our bodies is truly alarming. These tiny particles have been found in many parts of the human body, including the placenta, lungs, liver, urine, sputum, breast milk, blood, heart, and testicles. No part of your body is safe from this invasion.

And microplastics act as both physical and chemical threats. The physical aspect is easier to grasp at first. These tiny particles could block or inflame organisms that ingest them. But what's worse is that microplastics are like tiny, toxic sponges floating through your environment. They have an uncanny ability to absorb and concentrate other harmful chemicals that are also present in our water and soil. That means these tiny bits of plastic are carrying more than their own chemical load; they're also carrying a lot of other pollutants.

Here's where the true time-bomb aspect comes into play. The release of plastic toxins, especially xenoestrogens, isn't immediate. They activate your estrogen receptors and damage your mitochondria over time. It's a slow, gradual process that continues long after the microplastics have been ingested or absorbed. This means that the plastic pollution already created will continue to release harmful chemicals into the environment and our bodies for many generations to come, worsening every year.

What's more, this problem is cumulative. Every year, more plastic is produced and discarded. Every year, more of the existing plastic in the environment breaks down into micro- and nanoparticles. And every year, these particles absorb more toxins. It's a self-perpetuating cycle that feeds itself and grows more severe with each passing day. It's not just another environmental issue. This problem may soon overshadow many other concerns.

The long-term impact of microplastics on human health is a ticking time bomb. As these particles accumulate in your body over time, they slowly release their toxic payload. And it isn't a problem that will go away on its own. In fact, it's a problem that's set to worsen year after year, decade after decade.

Simple Steps to Reclaim Your Health from the Microplastics Menace
But it's not all doom and gloom. While the situation is dire, it's not hopeless. Awareness is growing, and with it, innovative solutions are emerging. Scientists and environmentalists are working hard to fix

this crisis. They are using biodegradable plastics and advanced filtration systems.

As individuals, we also have the power to make a difference. By reducing our plastic consumption, choosing sustainable alternatives, and supporting policies that address plastic pollution, we can start to turn the tide. It won't be easy, and it won't happen overnight, but it's a fight we can't afford to lose.

The story of plastics and microplastics is still unfolding, and it's up to us to write a healthier, safer ending. This isn't a problem with a simple solution. Other pollution often has specific sources that can be targeted, but microplastic pollution comes from our entire plastic-dependent way of life.

We must rethink our relationship with plastics. We must also change how we produce, consume, and dispose of plastic goods. It's a daunting task, but one that becomes more urgent with each passing year. Growing awareness and international efforts to curb plastic pollution offer a glimmer of hope. The challenge now lies in translating this awareness into effective action to stem the tide of plastic pollution.

Every positive action you take, no matter how small, compounds over time. Each plastic item you refuse, each sustainable choice you make, adds up. It's like making small, regular deposits into a savings account of planetary health. Over time, these actions may inspire others. They could spark a ripple effect of positive change.

In the face of such a monumental challenge, it's easy to feel overwhelmed. But remember, every journey begins with a single step. By educating yourself about the dangers of EDCs and microplastics, and by making conscious choices in your daily life, you're already making a difference. You have the power to protect your health and contribute to a cleaner, safer environment for future generations.

Microplastics are everywhere, but we can fight them. There are several strategies you can use that can greatly reduce your exposure to these harmful particles. Let's start with one of the most vital: water filtration. A high-quality water filter that removes microplastics is a major breakthrough. Look for filters with a fine pore size or those specifically designed to filter out these tiny particles. This simple step can cut your daily microplastic intake from drinking water.

Next, let's talk about containers. It's time to bid farewell to plastic and embrace alternatives. Use glass or stainless-steel water bottles instead of plastic ones. These materials shed no microplastics. They're also more durable and often prettier. The same goes for food storage—switch to glass containers. They're safer, don't absorb odors, and can even go from freezer to oven without a hitch.

When it comes to food packaging, a little caution goes a long way. Choose fresh, unwrapped produce over prepackaged items whenever possible. When buying packaged goods, select those in glass or cardboard rather than plastic. This not only reduces your microplastic exposure but often leads to healthier food choices.

Speaking of which, minimizing processed food consumption is another powerful strategy. These foods often come in plastic packaging and can contain higher levels of microplastics. Cooking at home with fresh ingredients cuts your exposure and boosts the quality of your nutrition.

Single-use plastics are a major contributor to the microplastic problem. Items like plastic cutlery, straws, and bags may seem convenient, but they come at a high cost to both your health and the environment. Make a conscious effort to reduce your use of these items. Carry reusable alternatives with you—a set of bamboo cutlery, a metal straw, a cloth shopping bag. These minor changes can make a substantial difference over time.

Your wardrobe choices can also impact your microplastic exposure. Synthetic fibers from clothing can shed microplastics during washing. Consider natural fabrics like cotton, wool, and silk whenever possible. When you do wash synthetic fabrics, use a laundry bag designed to capture microfibers. This simple step can prevent millions of plastic particles from entering our water systems with each wash.

Lastly, let's talk about cosmetics and personal care products. Many of these items contain microplastics, such as microbeads in scrub creams or glitter in makeup products. Scrutinize ingredient lists and opt for natural alternatives. Also, be wary of petroleum-based products. Not only can petroleum clog your pores, but it often contains harmful EDCs. Instead, try natural alternatives like lanolin. It's a wax from sheep's wool that mimics human sebum. It moisturizes even better than petroleum—with no risks.

In addition to switching from plastic to safer alternatives, perhaps the most meaningful change you can make is bidding farewell to all nonstick cookware. In its place, discover the joy of cooking with ceramic cookware and stainless-steel pots. Their gleaming surfaces are a testament to their durability and safety.

As you embrace these changes and become more aware, you'll notice a shift in your approach to consumption. You'll be drawn to products made from natural materials. Hardwood cutting boards, bamboo utensils and toothbrushes, beeswax food wraps, and cotton produce bags will be your new allies in your quest for an EDC-free life.

Each swap you make is a small victory, a step toward a healthier home environment. The change is stunning. Your shelves will shine with glass containers and the warm glow of natural materials. But beyond looks, you'll feel relieved. Your food won't touch EDC-leaching plastics.

The process isn't always easy. There will be some inconvenience and a longing for the simplicity of disposables. But with each meal prepared in your new cookware, each leftover stored in a glass container, you'll feel a growing sense of empowerment. You're not just avoiding EDCs; you're cultivating a more mindful, sustainable lifestyle.

Detox Strategies: Your Body's Defense Against EDCs

Reducing EDC exposure is crucial. But it's also vital to support your body's natural detox processes. One of the most effective ways to do this is to promote sweating. The heat from infrared or Finnish saunas can help release stored toxins by encouraging your body to sweat them out. Regular sauna use is also beneficial for those with heart or joint issues as well as for athletes looking to boost their performance.

Sauna heat works by causing stress that triggers beneficial adaptations, increasing nitric oxide in your blood vessels, activating heat-shock protein, prompting immune and hormonal changes, and inducing sweat to excrete toxins.

However, it's important to note that not all saunas are created equal. Many popular infrared saunas emit high levels of electromagnetic fields (EMFs). When choosing a sauna, find one that cuts EMF exposure and boosts detox. Exercise can also lower your tissue levels of EDCs by increasing sweat production. Therefore, combining exercise with sauna sessions can be very beneficial.

While sweating is an excellent way to release toxins, there's a catch. Once mobilized, these toxins can be reabsorbed in your intestines. That would put you right back where you started. This is where the importance of an effective binder comes into play.

By using a binder like activated charcoal, you can intercept these mobilized toxins before they have a chance to reenter your system. The key is in the timing: take about two grams of activated charcoal before your sauna and make sure that you're taking it at least one hour before and two hours after meals, supplements, or medications. This timing ensures the charcoal binds to the toxins and won't interfere with the absorption of your nutrients or medications.

Body Fat and EDCs: The Hidden Connection

As you navigate the world of environmental toxins, know this: many EDCs, including BPA/BPS, phthalates, PCBs, PBDEs, and pesticides, are fat-soluble. This characteristic means they tend to accumulate in your body fat. A low body-fat percentage cuts down space for unwanted guests. It's like giving EDCs fewer places to hide in your body.

This doesn't mean you need to strive for an unrealistically low body-fat percentage. Instead, focus on a diet made up of whole, unprocessed foods; avoid food that has been stored or cooked in plastic; and get regular exercise. This strategy fights EDCs, but it also improves health in many ways, boosting heart health, insulin sensitivity, and energy, to name a few.

It's important to note that EDCs make it harder to lose weight. If you struggle with shedding pounds, there might be biochemical reasons at play. The presence of EDCs in your body can interfere with your metabolism, making weight loss more challenging.

The Third E: EMFs—Understanding the Invisible World around Us

EMFs are the invisible force that surrounds all of us. They are everywhere. These fields encompass a wide spectrum of frequencies, ranging from the natural to the man-made. To truly grasp the impact of EMFs on your health, it's helpful to understand their nature and the various types you encounter daily.

Let's start with the natural sources of EMFs. Sunlight, the most familiar form of electromagnetic radiation, has been bathing our planet in its energy for billions of years. The Earth's magnetic field, a natural EMF source, protects us from cosmic radiation. It also helps many species navigate. These natural EMFs have always been present during human evolution, and our bodies have adapted to coexist with them.

However, the landscape of EMFs has changed dramatically in recent years. Synthetic sources of EMFs now dominate our environment. They include our home's wiring, our cell phones, and our office Wi-Fi routers. These artificial EMFs have added complexity to the electromagnetic environment, and your body is still struggling to adapt to them.

One crucial distinction among EMFs is the difference between pulsed and non-pulsed fields. Most man-made EMFs, including those from wireless devices, use alternating current (AC) and are pulsed. This means they rapidly switch on and off, creating a choppy, irregular pattern of electromagnetic energy. Your body operates on direct current (DC) and is more accustomed to the smooth, continuous non-pulsed EMFs found in nature.

This difference may explain why man-made EMFs are more disruptive than natural ones. After millions of years, your cells have evolved to respond to the gentle rhythms of natural EMFs. Now, they are suddenly bombarded by rapid bursts of electromagnetic energy. It's like trying to waltz to techno music—your body's natural rhythms are thrown into disarray.

Another important categorization of EMFs is the distinction between ionizing and nonionizing radiation. Ionizing radiation, like

X-rays and gamma rays, removes electrons from atoms and damages cells. The dangers of ionizing radiation are well known, and its use is strictly regulated in medicine and industry.

Nonionizing radiation includes radio waves, microwaves, and visible light. It is thought to be harmless. However, more recent research suggests nonionizing radiation has harmful effects. This is concerning because devices that emit nonionizing radiation are everywhere in your life.

The Flawed Foundation of Wireless Safety Standards

The current wireless safety standards, set by the Federal Communication Commission (FCC), are based on a measure called the Specific Absorption Rate, or SAR. The SAR is supposed to indicate the rate at which the body absorbs radio frequency (RF) energy. However, these standards have significant limitations that should give you pause.

First and foremost, the SAR is determined using a model based on a large adult male. This one-size-fits-all approach fails to account for the varying effects on women, children, and smaller individuals. It's like using a men's size 12 shoe as the standard for everyone—it simply doesn't fit the reality of human diversity.

Also, the SAR only measures the thermal effects of EMF exposure. It ignores any nonthermal biological impacts. We're potentially missing a huge part of the picture when it comes to EMF effects on human health.

Critics argue, and I agree, that these standards serve industry interests and do not protect public health. The telecom industry has taken a page from the tobacco industry's playbook, funding research to cast doubt on the link between EMF exposure and health issues.

They've even used the same PR agencies as Big Tobacco to hide the dangers of electromagnetic frequencies. As explained in chapter 1, highly tailored studies can be used to sow confusion and actively discredit anyone who reveals fraud.

Feeling Drained? Reverse the Hidden Impact of Magnetic and Electric Fields

When we talk about EMFs, we must distinguish between magnetic and electric fields. They affect your body in different ways. Magnetic fields, from electric currents, are concerning. They easily penetrate the human body. Many materials can block electric fields, but magnetic fields pass through most substances.

Research has linked prolonged exposure to strong magnetic fields to a higher risk of childhood leukemia and other health issues. This is worrying because many devices and appliances at home and work generate magnetic fields. From refrigerators to hair dryers, you are surrounded by magnetic fields that are silently harming your health.

Electric fields, on the other hand, can be more easily shielded. However, this doesn't mean they're harmless. Chronic exposure to electric fields also stresses your body—though they do not penetrate it as readily as magnetic fields. The key word here is chronic—it's the long-term, continuous exposure that we need to be concerned about.

Think about it this way: a single raindrop won't erode a rock, but constant dripping over time can carve a canyon. Similarly, brief exposure to electric fields might not cause any ill effects. But years of exposure could be significant. This is why it's crucial to consider not just the intensity of EMF exposure, but also its duration and frequency.

As we add more EMF-emitting devices to our lives, we're running a huge, uncontrolled experiment on ourselves. The long-term consequences of this experiment are yet to be fully understood, but the early signs are concerning. We must take EMF exposure seriously and protect ourselves and our loved ones from its potential harm.

The story of our increasing exposure to electromagnetic fields is a cautionary tale that begins with the discovery of X-rays in 1895. This new technology was quickly used for many things. These included processes that ranged from medical imaging to shoe fitting. At that time, its long-term health effects were not fully understood.

It's a classic case of technological enthusiasm outpacing scientific caution. Despite early indications of harmful effects, it took decades for proper regulations to be implemented. This history eerily parallels our situation with nonionizing EMFs. We often downplay potential risks in favor of technological progress.

As we entered the twentieth century, microwave technology increased EMF exposure. The microwave oven, based on radar technology, brought high-frequency EMFs into our homes. Suddenly, we were zapping our food with electromagnetic radiation. A few decades prior to its introduction, that would have seemed like science fiction. Microwave ovens made cooking easier, but they also added a new source of harmful EMF exposure that we still grapple with today.

The real explosion in personal EMF exposure came with cordless phones in the 1980s. Then, in the late 1990s and early 2000s, it was cell phones. These devices dramatically increased our daily exposure to EMFs. Think about it: we went from occasionally using a landline phone to carrying a powerful EMF-emitting device in our pockets all day, every day. The impact of this shift cannot be overstated. Today, there are more cell phones on the planet than there are people! We're essentially surrounded by a constant cloud of electromagnetic radiation.

But the EMF revolution didn't stop there. The rise of wireless internet and Wi-Fi in the late 1990s revolutionized connectivity. It also increased our EMF exposure. Wi-Fi routers are now in virtually every home, office, and public space, and they create a constant background of EMF radiation. The use of laptops, tablets, and smartphones has also radically increased.

Recent studies show the typical internet user spends 6 hours and 40 minutes online each day. That's 46.7 hours a week. That's nearly six times the online time spent at the turn of the century. We're bathing in EMFs for more than a quarter of our day!

Our EMF level of exposure is already concerning, but 5G technology will raise it even more. The 5G technology offers faster internet and better connectivity, but it raises new issues about EMF exposure because this technology needs a denser network of antennas.

The Internet of Things (IoT), a network of smart devices, combined with the 5G network, will greatly increase EMF levels in our environment. We're talking about a world where our phones, fridges, cars, and clothes are always sending and receiving signals. And they're all electromagnetic.

To grasp our rising EMF exposure, consider this: You are now exposed to 1 billion-billion times more EMFs than we were a century ago. That's not a typo—it has 10 with 18 zeros after it. When I share this statistic in my lectures, no one ever guesses correctly. Most people estimate an increase of 10 to 1,000 times, with the occasional brave soul venturing a guess of a million times. But even these seemingly outrageous guesses fall far short of the reality. We've gone from living in a world with minimal man-made EMFs to one that's saturated with them in just a century—a blink of an eye in evolutionary terms.

The health implications of this increased EMF exposure are a subject of ongoing research and debate. The acute effects of high-level EMF exposure are well known. But the long-term effects of chronic, low-level exposure to many EMF sources are unclear. However, strong research links EMF exposure to various health issues. These include sleep disturbances, hormonal imbalances, and even certain types of cancer. These effects, like the effects of smoking, often develop slowly over time, so it may be hard to link them to EMF exposure. That's why long-term, large-scale studies are so important in this field.

I recall one of my friends, Karliin, who had been suffering from chronic insomnia and fatigue for years. After we found high EMF levels in her bedroom from a nearby cell tower, she shielded it. Within weeks, her sleep quality improved significantly. Stories like this underscore the importance of being proactive about EMF exposure.

Practical Steps to Minimize EMF Exposure in Your Daily Life
Let's talk about those wireless devices we all love. Your smartphone, tablet, and laptop are your constant companions, but they're also constant EMF emitters. The key to safety is distance. Keep these devices away from your body as much as possible. When you're not actively

using them, store them in another room or, better yet, in a Faraday bag. And please, for the love of your health, stop sleeping with your phone under your pillow!

Creating low-EMF zones in your living spaces is another crucial step. Your bedroom should be your EMF sanctuary. After all, you spend about a third of your life there. Remove all unnecessary electronics. Use battery-powered alarm clocks. Consider installing an EMF kill switch to cut power to the room at night. Trust me, your sleep quality will improve dramatically.

When it comes to your computer setup, wired is the way to go. Replace that wireless mouse and keyboard with wired versions. Use a grounded power cord for your laptop and connect to the internet with a grounded Ethernet cable. If you must use Wi-Fi, disable it on your router and devices when it's not in use. Every little bit helps in reducing your overall EMF exposure.

Your cell phone is likely your biggest source of personal EMF exposure. Here's a radical idea: use it less. When you do use it, put it on speakerphone or use an air-tube headset to keep it away from your head. Avoid using your phone in areas with weak signals. It must work harder in these areas, emitting more EMFs. And for goodness' sake, stop carrying it in your pocket! Use a bag or purse instead, keeping that EMF generator away from your vital organs.

Replace metal bed frames and spring mattresses with non-metal alternatives. Metal acts as an antenna for EMFs, amplifying your exposure while you sleep. The bed I use doesn't even have metal screws in it. It is all wood.

Have your bedside lamps rewired with shielded cords to further minimize electric fields. Remember, never leave your cell phone overnight on your nightstand. And please, ditch that electric blanket. The EMFs it generates so close to your body all night long are just not worth the warmth.

Here's another tip that might surprise you: minimize your use of fluorescent and LED bulbs. While they're energy-efficient, they generate significant amounts of dirty electricity (see below). Use incandescent bulbs in areas where you spend a lot of time. Yes, they use more energy, but they're much cleaner from an EMF perspective.

When you do use LED bulbs, be sure to only use the warm versions as the brighter versions have far too much blue light that can disrupt your circadian rhythm.

Tackling Indoor Magnetic Fields and Dirty Electricity

We all live with sneaky indoor magnetic fields. They're everywhere, from your microwave to your hair dryer. Start by using a gauss meter to identify problem areas in your home. You might be surprised at what you find. Once you've identified the culprits, address any wiring issues and keep your distance from appliances with motors.

Be particularly cautious of circuit breaker boxes. I've seen many cases where people's health improved after moving their bed or workspace away from EMF hotspots. I even realized the headboard of my bed shares a common wall with my garage. The charger for my electric car was literally a few feet from my head, so I learned never to charge my car overnight while I was sleeping.

Dirty electricity is another often-overlooked source of EMFs in your home. This electromagnetic noise travels along your home's wiring, creating a pervasive field of EMFs. Installing dirty-electricity filters can help clean up this electromagnetic pollution. Consider whole-house filtering systems for comprehensive protection.

If you have solar power like I do, pay attention to the placement of your inverters. These generate significant magnetic fields. There are 20 KHz filters you can professionally install in them to remove this source of dirty electricity.

Tackling External EMF Sources: Your First Line of Defense

When it comes to EMF exposure, your home is your castle, but even castles need proper fortification. Let's start with the external threats. Power lines, those ubiquitous conductors of electricity, are a significant source of EMFs. If you're house hunting, pay close attention to nearby power lines. The closer you are, the higher your exposure. I've seen patients whose health improved after moving away from high-voltage power lines.

Before you sign that lease or purchase agreement, grab an EMF meter and do a thorough sweep of the property. You might be surprised at what you find. I once had a patient who was experiencing chronic fatigue and headaches. When we measured the EMF levels in her new apartment, we discovered it was riddled with hotspots from the building's electrical system. Knowledge is power—and in this case, it can also be the key to your health.

Be particularly wary of homes and apartments with electric radiant heat. These systems create a pervasive EMF field throughout your living space. If you're already in such a place, consider using EMF-blocking mats under your bed and in areas where you spend a lot of time. It's not a perfect solution, but it can significantly reduce your EMF exposure.

Smart utility meters are another modern convenience that comes with a hefty EMF price tag. If possible, opt out of having one installed in your home. If that's not an option, invest in a smart-meter guard. These simple devices can reduce the EMF emissions from your meter by up to 98 percent. It's a small step that can make a substantial difference in your exposure.

Shielding Techniques: Your EMF Armor

Sometimes, despite your best efforts, EMFs still find their way into your living space. That's where extra shielding techniques come into play. Think of it as putting on armor before heading into battle—except in this case, the battle is against invisible electromagnetic waves.

Start with your windows. They're like open doors for EMFs. Install RF-blocking window treatments; these can be curtains, films, or even specially designed blinds. They not only block EMFs but can also help with temperature regulation, potentially lowering your energy bills. It's a win-win situation. EMF-blocking paint can also help block high-frequency signals.

For your portable devices, Faraday bags are a game changer. These simple pouches act like a force field, blocking all incoming and outgoing signals. I always keep my phone in a Faraday bag when I'm not using it. It's an effortless way to give your body a break from constant EMF bombardment.

I know what you're thinking: "But Dr. Mercola, I can't live in a Faraday cage!" And you're right. If you need to go into high-EMF areas, consider EMF-protective clothing. From underwear to outerwear, there are now garments designed to shield your body from EMFs. It might sound extreme, but in our increasingly wireless world, it's becoming a necessary precaution.

EMF Meters: Your Eyes in the Electromagnetic Storm

You wouldn't try to navigate a ship through stormy seas without proper instruments, would you? Well, navigating our EMF-saturated world without an EMF meter is just as risky. Investing in a quality EMF meter is one of the best decisions you can make for your health.

There's something profoundly impactful about hearing the invisible culprits. EMF meters with sound feedback make electromagnetic fields more real. It's like suddenly gaining a new sense—electromagnetic hearing, if you will.

As you move through your home with an EMF meter, the quiet atmosphere suddenly comes alive with beeps, crackles, and whines. That gentle ping near your bedside lamp grows to an urgent wail as you approach your cell-phone charger. Your smart TV emits a constant hum, while your microwave oven screams with activity when in use. It's a startling revelation. Your body and brain are always bathed in a cacophony of electromagnetic "noise" you never knew existed.

This audio trip through your EMF landscape shows your daily exposure. It's a wake-up call, transforming abstract concerns into measurable phenomena. Suddenly, creating a quieter electromagnetic environment becomes a tangible goal.

Learning to use an EMF meter yourself is empowering. It allows you to take control of your environment and identify hidden EMF sources that you might otherwise miss. I remember the first time I used an EMF meter in my own home. I was shocked to discover a significant EMF hotspot right where I used to sit and read every evening. A simple rearrangement of furniture made a world of difference for me.

Once you've identified the EMF sources in your environment, you can work on your mitigation efforts. Focus on the areas where you spend the most time—your bedroom, your home office, and your favorite reading nook. Remember, when it comes to EMFs, every little bit of reduction helps.

The Fourth E: Endotoxins—Your Silent Saboteurs

The energy production impairment created by the first three Es—vegetable and seed oils, estrogen, and EMFs—causes damage to well over 99.9 percent of us. The most serious result is that it limits your ability to evacuate oxygen from the large bowel. This then causes a shift from predominantly beneficial oxygen-intolerant bacteria to oxygen-tolerant pathogenic or disease-causing bacteria in your gut.

The dominance of oxygen-tolerant bacteria in your gut isn't just a minor imbalance—it's a serious health concern. These bacteria produce endotoxins that are far more potent and harmful than those made by their oxygen-intolerant counterparts. As a result, if your gut microbiome has too many oxygen-tolerant species, you likely have high endotoxin levels. And trust me, your body can't handle this easily. It's especially true when your cellular energy production is already low.

So, let's talk about these endotoxins. They're essentially waste products released when bad bacteria die, but they are also powerful inflammatory agents. Endotoxins trigger both acute and chronic inflammation, and they're implicated in a wide range of diseases. We're talking about serious conditions: leaky gut, Alzheimer's, Parkinson's, heart attacks, and sepsis. But it doesn't stop there. Recent studies have shown that endotoxins also contribute to anxiety and depression.

The Cascade of Endotoxin Effects

When endotoxins make their way into your tissues, they set off a cascade of events with far-reaching consequences for your health. Their first target? Your mitochondria. The erosion caused by endotoxins slowly reduces your mitochondria's ability to produce vital energy, which fuels every process in your body.

This creates a downward spiral. As your mitochondria falter, unable to keep up with the demands of the body, a ripple effect spreads throughout your gut. Oxygen begins to seep into what was an oxygen-free sanctuary. The oxygen-tolerant pathogenic bacteria start to multiply.

Gut bacteria double in population every three to sixteen hours. If not addressed, this can quickly cause chronic digestive discomfort.

Their numbers grow as they feast on the newfound abundance of oxygen in the gut. As they do so, they crowd out the oxygen-intolerant bacteria, and a new, harmful balance of power emerges. The result is systemic inflammation, as your body's immune system goes on high alert, attacking these foreign invaders.

Your Gut Microbiome Is Likely in Chaos

As this process unfolds, your gut microbiome undergoes dramatic changes. The once oxygen-free environment of your gut becomes increasingly oxygenated. This shift creates a perfect breeding ground for oxygen-tolerant bacteria, which will then begin to thrive and multiply in your gut.

These opportunistic bacteria quickly take over the gut. They crowd out the beneficial, oxygen-intolerant species that once dominated and profoundly alter your gut's terrain. The prevailing bacteria now produce harmful endotoxins, worsening inflammation and damaging your mitochondria.

This altered gut environment also decreases the production of beneficial compounds. These include short-chain fatty acids (SCFAs), which help maintain gut health, support your immune system, and have a positive effect on your mood and mental health.

The implications of this gut microbiome chaos extend far beyond digestive discomfort. It affects your health, energy levels, mental clarity, and even your susceptibility to various diseases. That's why I always emphasize the importance of maintaining a healthy gut environment. It's not just about digestive health—it's about whole-body wellness.

Let me break it down for you. When endotoxins make their way into your gut, they don't just float around harmlessly. They're on a mission, and their target is a specific protein called the TLR-4 (toll-like receptor 4). This receptor is like a sentinel on your gut's cellular walls, always on the lookout for potential threats. When endotoxins bind to these receptors, it's like setting off a cellular alarm system.

The moment this binding occurs, your gut cells go into panic mode. They start pumping out pro-inflammatory cytokines and chemokines like there's no tomorrow. These inflammatory molecules act like tiny wrecking balls. They slowly chip away at the tight junctions between your gut cells. These tight junctions are neces-sary because they're what keep the contents of your gut where they belong, inside your digestive tract. As these junctions weaken, your gut becomes more permeable, causing the "leaky" gut condition that is at the root of countless health issues.

The Vicious Cycle: A Downward Spiral of Health

As your exposure to endotoxins increases, there is more damage to your gut and mitochondria. This can come from a poor diet, environ-mental toxins, or other factors. This damage makes you even more vulnerable to the effects of endotoxins. Your gut becomes leakier, allowing more endotoxins to enter your bloodstream. Your mitochon-dria become less efficient, making it harder for your body to deal with these toxins.

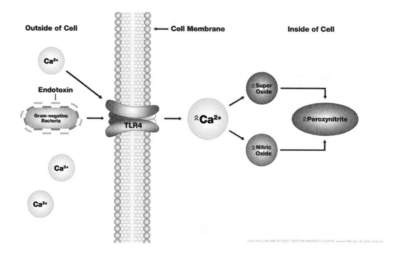

Endotoxin-Induced Cellular Signaling and Oxidative Stress: This diagram illustrates the cascade of events triggered by gram-negative bacterial endotoxins at the cellular level.

It's a downward spiral that leads to the epidemic of chronic health disease most of us are experiencing. I've seen it contribute to everything from autoimmune diseases to neurodegenerative disorders. The real tragedy is that conventional medicine misses this cause and focuses on treating symptoms instead.

But here's the good news: once you understand this cycle, you can take steps to break it. You can reverse this damage and reclaim your health by reducing your exposure to endotoxins and protecting your mitochondria.

In the unabridged version of this book, complete with references, I review the complex biology of how endotoxins, LA, EDCs, and EMFs all share a similar biological pathway. It ultimately increases free-radical damage, but not through the normal reactive oxygen species. Instead, it's through a reactive nitrogen species called peroxynitrite that you have likely never heard of.

So, let's break down exactly what peroxynitrite does to your cells. First off, it's a long-lasting reactive species. Unlike some other free radicals that disappear quickly, peroxynitrite sticks around, giving it more time to do damage.

One of peroxynitrite's favorite targets is your cell membranes. It causes lipid peroxidation, which is a fancy way of saying it pokes holes in the walls of your cells. Imagine trying to keep your house warm in the winter with Swiss cheese for walls. That's what peroxynitrite does to your cells.

But it doesn't stop there. Peroxynitrite also damages proteins and DNA. It's like a bull in a china shop, breaking and twisting crucial cellular components. This can lead to enzyme dysfunction, gene mutations, and a host of other problems.

The effects of peroxynitrite aren't limited to one area of your body. It can cause damage to your cardiovascular system, leading to atherosclerosis. In your lungs, it can trigger inflammation and oxidative damage. It interferes with insulin signaling, potentially contributing to diabetes. In your brain it's been linked to neurodegenerative diseases like Alzheimer's and Parkinson's.

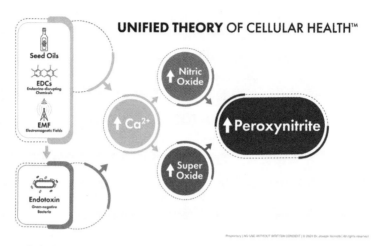

The Unified Theory of Cellular Health™ diagram illustrates the interconnected pathways leading to cellular stress. It shows how environmental factors like seed oils, endocrine-disrupting chemicals (EDCs), and electromagnetic fields (EMFs) can synergize with endotoxins from gram-negative bacteria to elevate intracellular calcium levels (Ca2+).

Carbon Dioxide: The Misunderstood Key to Getting Your Life Back

An unexpected ally in the fight against peroxynitrite is carbon dioxide. Your body produces it naturally. That's right—the same CO_2 you breathe out is a potent defender against oxidative stress.

When CO_2 combines with peroxynitrite, it creates a new compound that's far less reactive and damaging than peroxynitrite. It's like turning a raging fire into a smoldering ember. This reaction effectively neutralizes the threat, giving your cells a chance to repair and recover from oxidative damage.

The implications of this are huge. Keeping therapeutic CO_2 levels in your body creates a natural buffer against oxidative damage from peroxynitrite. It's a prime example of how your body has evolved to use clever defense mechanisms—we just need to support them properly.

So, how can you put this knowledge into action? There are several strategies you can use to increase your body's CO_2 levels and protect against peroxynitrite damage.

First, consider incorporating specific breathing techniques into your daily routine. Techniques like Buteyko and box breathing can slightly raise your CO_2 levels. This can help protect you. I've had patients report significant gains in energy and clarity after using these techniques.

Diet and exercise also play an important role. Eating a diet rich in antioxidants and engaging in regular physical activity can help your body produce and use CO_2 more efficiently.

For over a year, I've been developing a new strategy that involves safely introducing carbon dioxide gas directly into the colon. This may sound unusual or concerning at first. But it's important to note that gastroenterologists have been using CO_2 gas in the colon during colonoscopies for twenty-five years. This established medical practice provides a foundation of safety for our innovative approach.

While I'm still fine-tuning the details of this therapy, I'm incredibly excited about its potential. Based on my research and preliminary results, I believe this could be one of the most significant breakthroughs we've seen in gut health and overall wellness. The implications for healing and maintaining a healthy microbiome are profound.

I understand you might have questions or want to stay updated on this developing therapy. That's why I've set up a system to keep you informed. If you download the Coach app, I'll be able to send you updates as soon as they're available. This way, you'll be among the first to know when this therapy is ready for wider use.

This CO_2 therapy isn't just another supplement or diet plan. I truly believe it has the potential to be a game-changer in our approach to gut health and, by extension, your total health. As I've discussed throughout this book, the state of your gut affects every aspect of your well-being. By directly addressing gut health in this novel way, we may be opening doors to levels of gut improvement that were previously out of reach.

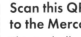 **Scan this QR code to get FREE access to the Mercola Health Coach app.** This tool allows you to log your meals, track your macronutrient ratios, and monitor your progress over time.

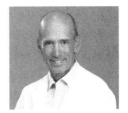

CHAPTER 5

Let Sunlight Gently Guide and Brighten Your Journey Back to Health

Picture yourself sitting in a grand cosmic theater, with the sun taking center stage. It's not just putting on a light show—it's the star of the whole energy production for life on Earth. As you watch this celestial performance, you'll start to see how this amazing ball of fire in the sky connects everything and everyone, including you.

Now, let's zoom in on the real heroes of this story: electrons. These tiny particles are like the delivery trucks of the energy world. They're constantly moving around, carrying energy from one place to another. When an electron is energized, it jumps up to a higher level. When it comes back down, it releases that energy, like a fireworks display on a microscopic scale.

This electron dance is happening all around us, all the time. It's how plants turn sunlight into food through photosynthesis. The sun zaps electrons in the plant's chlorophyll, and those excited electrons trigger a chain reaction that creates the energy the plant needs to grow.

But it's not just plants that enjoy this electron shuffle. Your smartphone, your TV, even the lights in your house all work due to the

130

movement of electrons. When you plug something in, you're basically giving those electrons a track to run on. And in your own body, every single cell is using electrons to create the energy it needs to keep you going.

So next time you're soaking up some rays, remember you're not just getting a tan. You're plugging into the ultimate power source of life on Earth!

The Unexpected Truth About Sunlight That Can Give You Your Life Back

For more than thirty years, I've been shouting from the rooftops about how important sunlight is for our health. It's been my passion, my mission, to help people understand that the sun isn't our enemy— it's one of our best friends when it comes to staying healthy. And now, finally, the tide is turning.

Back in the day, doctors used to prescribe sunbathing as a cure for all sorts of ailments. Then the pendulum swung the other way. Suddenly, we were told to hide from the sun like vampires. We had to slather on sunscreen every time we stepped outside. But here's the thing: that advice was missing a big piece of the puzzle.

Recent studies, especially large ones from Sweden and the UK, show that more sun exposure is linked to longer life and lower risk of heart disease. This means the very thing we've been told to avoid might actually help us live longer, healthier lives.

And it's not just about longevity. During the COVID-19 pandemic, researchers noticed that areas with more sunlight had fewer severe cases. You might be thinking, "But Dr. Mercola, isn't this all just about vitamin D?" That's part of it, but it's not the whole story. Sunlight does more for your body than just help you make vitamin D. For example, it triggers your skin to produce nitric oxide. This can lower your blood pressure. It also helps regulate your sleep-wake cycle and even influences how your brain and body work.

Here's a fascinating tidbit: over thousands of years, people living far from the equator developed lighter skin. Why? To soak up more of that precious sunlight in locations where it wasn't as strong. It's as if our bodies knew how important sun exposure was and adapted to make the most of it.

But here's where it gets tricky: the benefits of sun exposure can vary depending on your skin color. If you have darker skin, you might need more time in the sun to get the same benefits as someone with lighter skin. This is why we need to move away from one-size-fits-all advice about sun exposure and start thinking about what's right for you.

Let's talk about how your body turns sunlight into vitamin D. It's like a mini factory in your skin, and it's pretty amazing when you think about it. When the sun's ultraviolet B (UVB) rays hit your skin, they kick off a chain reaction. Your skin has a substance called 7-dehydrocholesterol. When UVB rays hit it, it turns into pre-vitamin D3. Then, your body quickly converts that into vitamin D3, which is the form your body can use.

Vitamin D3 is required for so many things in your body. It keeps your bones strong by helping you absorb calcium. But that's just the beginning. Research shows that enough vitamin D can reduce your risk of many health problems, from multiple sclerosis to some cancers. It's like a health insurance policy that you can get just by stepping outside.

The catch is, making vitamin D isn't as simple as just being in the sun. Many factors affect how much vitamin D your body produces. For example, the time of year matters—in the winter, the sun's rays aren't as strong. Where you live on the planet is important too. If you're farther from the equator, the sun's rays must travel through more atmosphere to reach you. Both of these factors can reduce the sun's potential to help your body produce vitamin D.

Your age is another consideration. As you get older, your skin doesn't produce vitamin D as efficiently as it used to. Coverings like sunscreen and clothes also play a role. They can block the UV rays that cause sunburn, but they also reduce your skin's ability to make vitamin D.

Not getting enough vitamin D can lead to some serious problems. In kids, it can cause rickets, which makes bones soft and weak. In adults, it can lead to a condition called osteomalacia, which is basically adult rickets. Beyond bone health, vitamin D deficiency has been linked to an increased risk of heart disease and autoimmune disorders.

You might be thinking, "No problem, I'll just take a vitamin D supplement." However, while supplements can be helpful, they're not quite the same as getting your vitamin D from the sun. Sunlight triggers other beneficial processes in your skin that we're still learning about. It's similar to the difference between eating an orange and taking a vitamin C pill—the orange has a lot of other good stuff in it that the pill just can't replicate.

The takeaway is, supplements have their place, but nothing beats good old-fashioned sunshine for getting vitamin D. It's about balance. We need enough sun to be healthy, but too much sun exposure can result in getting sunburn and skin cancer.

In my years of studying this, I've come to see sunlight as an essential nutrient, just like the vitamins and minerals we get from food. Your body is designed to use sunlight and to thrive on it. So don't be afraid of the sun. Respect it, use it wisely, and let it help you be the healthiest version of yourself you can be.

Supplementing Vitamin D Wisely: When Sunshine Isn't Enough

While getting your vitamin D from sunlight is ideal, it's not always possible. If you live in a northern climate, work indoors, or have darker skin, you may need vitamin D supplements. But before you rush out to buy vitamin D pills, there are a few things to consider.

First, it's important to understand that vitamin D doesn't work alone. It's part of a complex interplay of nutrients in your body. When supplementing with vitamin D, you also need to pay attention to your intake of magnesium, calcium, and vitamin K2. These nutrients work synergistically, and imbalances can occur if one is taken in isolation at high doses. This is why calcium supplements may raise the risk of heart attack and stroke. They're often taken without enough vitamin D and K2.

I've seen the importance of this balance in my practice. One patient, John, came to me with muscle cramps and fatigue. He had been taking high doses of vitamin D, and although our nutrient test showed his vitamin D was high, his magnesium was very low. After we added magnesium and cut his vitamin D, his symptoms improved substantially.

The most reliable way to know your vitamin D status is regular testing. Having this information can also help determine the correct supplement dosage. I recommend getting your levels checked at least twice a year. Once you know your current vitamin D levels, you can adjust your sun exposure or vitamin D3 supplementation accordingly. It's a good idea to retest after three to four months to confirm that you've reached and are maintaining the desired vitamin D level.

Remember, while supplements can be helpful, they fall short of replicating the full spectrum of benefits derived from natural sunlight. Whenever possible, try to get your vitamin D the way nature intended—from the sun. When that's not workable, smart supplementation can help. It should be guided by regular tests and balanced with other nutrients to ensure you get the vitamin D your body needs to thrive.

In my years of practice, I've seen the power of optimizing vitamin D levels, whether through sun exposure or careful supplements. It can transform people. From improved mood and sleep to stronger bones and a more robust immune system, the benefits are truly remarkable. So, whether you're in the sun or taking a supplement, you're giving your body a powerful tool. It's key to achieving and maintaining optimal health.

Sunlight: The Key to Recovering Your Health and Increasing Longevity

Let me tell you about a groundbreaking study from Sweden that's going to change the way you think about sunlight. For years, "experts" have been telling you to avoid the sun as if it were your sworn enemy. But this research turns that idea on its head. A study followed a large group of women for two decades and found that those who avoided the sun had a much higher risk of dying at an earlier age. In contrast, those who soaked up the rays regularly had a lower risk.

In fact, the impact of avoiding sun exposure on your life expectancy is comparable to smoking. You heard that right—hiding from the sun could shorten your life as much as lighting up a cigarette! Sun-avoiders had a life expectancy up to two years shorter than those who got the most sun exposure.

Observational studies have also shown that people who get more sun exposure tend to live longer than those who are less exposed. In one study, sunseekers were 14 percent less likely to die from any cause over the course of thirteen years of follow-up compared to those who avoided the sun. Their risk of dying specifically from heart disease was 19 percent lower than the sun avoiders.

These findings challenge the oversimplified notion that sun exposure should be avoided at all costs. Yes, excessive sun exposure and the subsequent sunburn are harmful. But moderate sun exposure may have great health benefits. It's all about finding the right balance.

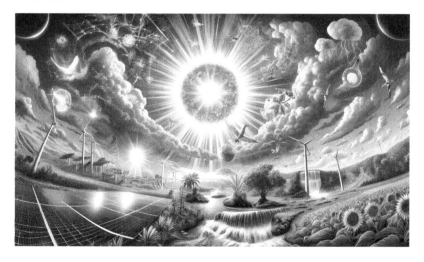

The Sun as the Universal Source of Electrons in Nature and Technology. This artwork encapsulates the concept that the sun's provision of electrons is the common thread linking all forms of life and technology. It presents a unifying vision of our world, where the fundamental processes of nature—from photosynthesis to human cellular metabolism, and the pinnacle of human innovation—are all traced back to the same stellar origin: the electron-emitting power of our sun.

Picture this: you have a beautiful philodendron plant sitting on your windowsill. It seems content enough, but it's not thriving. But imagine planting that same philodendron outdoors, where it gets full, unfiltered sunlight. Fast-forward a few years, and you'd hardly recognize it. It would have exploded in size, with leaves and stems that remind you of prehistoric flora. The secret to this incredible transformation is sunlight, plain and simple.

This analogy perfectly illustrates how sunlight acts as an unrecognized nutrient for our bodies. Just like that indoor plant, many of us are surviving on the limited "sunlight" that filters through our windows, but we're not truly thriving. Did you know that Americans spend about 87 percent of their time indoors and another 6 percent in enclosed vehicles? That's a whopping 93 percent of our time cut off from direct sunlight. No wonder we're seeing such widespread vitamin D deficiency and related health issues!

In addition to vitamin D production, sunlight is a key player in activating other essential nutrients in our bodies. Take vitamin A, for example. Sunlight allows vitamin A to be converted into its active form, retinoids, which are almost as important to maintaining good health as vitamin D. These compounds are vital for immune function, vision, and cell growth.

And here's something that might surprise you: sunlight even impacts your testosterone levels. If you get enough sun exposure and have a surplus of cellular energy, it can increase your testosterone production. You might think, "But Dr. Mercola, isn't testosterone just for men?" Not at all! While men do have and need more testosterone than women, it's an important hormone for women too. It plays a role in muscle mass, bone density, and even libido for both sexes.

Harnessing the Sun's Energy to Increase Your Energy

Here's something really exciting: your body can harness energy directly from the sun. You might think, "Wait a minute, I'm not a plant. I can't photosynthesize!" While you can't produce glucose from sunlight like plants do, your body has evolved to use sunlight in amazing ways.

Everything that keeps you going—every breath, every heartbeat, every thought—ultimately depends on the sun. When you eat a piece of fruit or a vegetable, you're consuming energy that the plant captured from the sun. When you eat meat, you're consuming energy from an animal that ate plants (or ate other animals that ate plants). It all traces back to the sun.

Your body has an incredible system for turning the food you eat into usable energy, and it all happens at the cellular level. It starts with digestion, when your body breaks down food into smaller parts. These parts then go through something called the Krebs cycle, which is like a cellular energy factory. From there, electrons move into the mitochondrial electron transport chain—and this is where the magic happens. The electron transport chain takes those electrons and turns them into ATP, which is like cellular fuel.

Incidentally, I've been working on studies that suggest our bodies might be able to do something similar to photosynthesis. I call it "photometabolism." Essentially, it means our bodies can take energy directly from the sun and turn it into electrons that feed our electron transport chain, just like the electrons from food do. It's a revolutionary concept that could change how we think about energy production in the human body.

But sometimes things go haywire in this process. When there are too many electrons floating around, it can cause something called reductive stress. It's like a traffic jam in your cells. This blockage happens for a couple of reasons. Sometimes, the flow of electrons through the electron transport chain gets gummed up. Other times, your body might be making too many electron carriers (molecules called NADH and FADH2), causing a backup.

One common cause of reductive stress is not getting enough carbohydrates. Your body typically needs about 250 grams of carbs a day to efficiently make energy. When you don't meet this quota, your body instead burns fat. This process cranks up the production of FADH2, which leads to that cellular traffic jam we mentioned previously.

When electrons get stuck, they can react with oxygen, which creates harmful compounds called reactive oxygen species (ROS). These troublemakers can wreak havoc on your body, causing inflammation and other health issues.

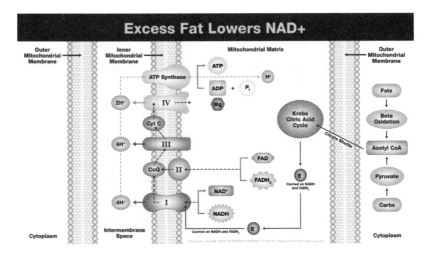

The Mitochondrial Electron Transport Chain and ATP Synthesis. This illustration shows the relationship between electron transport, proton pumping, and ATP production in mitochondrial energy metabolism. The image depicts the inner structure of a mitochondrion, showing the outer and inner mitochondrial membranes, the intermembrane space, and the mitochondrial matrix.

How to Resolve Reductive Stress Once It Happens

Reductive stress can make you feel less than your best, which is why it's important to fuel yourself with sufficient carbs to avert this molecular crisis. If it has already happened, don't worry, though—there's a solution! Grounding, or earthing, is a simple way to help your body get rid of those extra electrons. The idea is that by connecting your body directly to the earth, you can let those surplus electrons flow out of you and into the ground. It's as if your body is an electrical device and the earth is a giant battery that can absorb any excess charge.

One of the best and easiest ways to do this is to simply walk barefoot on the earth or lie down on the ground and let your skin touch the soil or grass. You can also submerge yourself in water, such as a lake or the ocean. These activities help to "ground" you, or electrically reconnect you to the earth.

However, if you live in North America, there's a problem. In many places, the electrical power that comes into our homes and buildings is full of distortions and interference caused by modern electrical devices such as computers, cell-phone chargers, and energy-efficient lighting. This "dirty electricity" can make it harder for your body to connect to the earth and release those extra electrons.

But there's one place where you can still get a good grounding: the ocean. The ocean is like a giant grounding pad because it's so vast and conductive. When you immerse yourself in seawater, your body becomes part of this huge, electrically conductive environment, and it's much easier for those surplus electrons to flow out of you.

Think of it like this: When you build up a static charge from walking around on a carpeted floor, you get a shock when you touch a doorknob, right? That's because the doorknob is grounded, and it allows the excess electrons to flow out of your body. Grounding in the ocean is like that but on a much bigger scale.

So, if you're feeling a little out of balance or if you think you might have some reductive stress going on, try to find some time to connect with the earth. Walk barefoot on the grass, lie down on the sand, or take a dip in the ocean. Let those excess electrons flow out of you and feel your body coming back into balance.

Alternatives to Safe Grounding in North America

If you live in North America and aren't lucky enough to be close to the ocean, don't lose heart. There's a safe and inexpensive medicinal solution that can help. Now, I know you might think,"I thought you weren't a fan of drugs, Dr. Mercola!" And you're right; I'm generally not. But the drug I'm talking about is different. Methylene blue has the distinction of being the very first synthesized drug—way back in 1876. German chemists originally developed it as an industrial dye for coloring textiles, particularly that vibrant blue color in blue jeans. But they quickly realized that methylene blue had a lot more to offer.

In the late nineteenth century, scientists discovered that methylene blue had some impressive medical properties. It became the first synthetic compound used as a malaria medication. Fast-forward to today and you'll find methylene blue being used in emergency rooms all around the world for a variety of critical applications. One of its main uses is for treating methemoglobinemia, a condition where hemoglobin can't release oxygen effectively to the body tissues. It's also used as an antidote for certain types of poisonings, like cyanide poisoning, carbon monoxide exposure, and cocaine overdose.

Methylene blue also has powerful metabolic benefits. It's an electron acceptor, which means it can temporarily remove the bottleneck of electrons created by faulty metabolism. Here's how it works: when methylene blue removes the surplus electrons that are clogging up the electron transport chain in your mitochondria, it allows your mitochondria to start producing cellular energy again. It's not a cure, but it can serve as a powerful crutch to support your metabolism while you're working to repair the underlying causes.

If you live by the ocean, you don't need to worry about using methylene blue because the ocean can naturally drain your surplus electrons through grounding. But if you're not near the ocean, methylene blue can be a great alternative.

Avoid Using Methylene Blue Solutions

The one caveat is to make sure you're only using pharmaceutical-grade methylene blue in capsule or tablet form and only as prescribed by a health-care professional. Many people choose to consume liquid formulas of methylene blue. However, dissolving methylene blue in water leads to a significant decrease in its effectiveness after forty-eight to seventy-two hours for several reasons:

1. **Photodegradation**. Methylene blue is sensitive to light, particularly UV radiation. When exposed to natural or artificial light, the chemical structure of methylene blue breaks down, resulting in a loss of therapeutic properties. This degradation process is accelerated when the compound is dissolved in water and exposed to light, diminishing its effectiveness.

2. **Chemical reactions**. In aqueous solutions, methylene blue can undergo redox reactions, especially in the presence of other substances that may act as reducing agents. These reactions can alter the chemical structure of methylene blue, reducing its ability to function effectively as a medication.

3. **Adsorption to container surfaces**. Methylene blue molecules can adsorb onto the surfaces of the container in which they

are stored, such as glass or plastic. This adsorption reduces the concentration of methylene blue available in the solution, effectively decreasing the dosage that can be administered.

4. **Instability in aqueous solutions**. Methylene blue tends to be less stable in water compared to its powdered form. The aqueous environment facilitates interactions between methylene blue and other dissolved substances, which might lead to precipitation or the formation of less active complexes.

5. **Increased risk of contamination**. Solutions of methylene blue, once prepared, are more susceptible to bacterial contamination compared to solid forms. Contamination can further degrade the solution or lead to the production of by-products that diminish its effectiveness and pose safety risks.

For these reasons, I only recommend using pharmaceutical-grade methylene blue in capsule or tablet form, not premixed liquids, and only as prescribed by a health-care professional.

How to Use Methylene Blue

Selecting the correct quality grade is important. There are three types typically sold—industrial grade, chemical grade (laboratory grade), and pharmaceutical grade. Industrial grade is the one typically sold in pet stores as aquarium cleaner. The only one you should use is the pharmaceutical grade. Industrial- and laboratory-grade methylene blue contain impurities and should never be used for medicinal purposes, including pet care.

Pharmaceutical-grade methylene blue is a prescription drug and can only legally be used with a prescription from a doctor. While you can easily and cheaply purchase methylene blue online, these products are rarely pharmaceutical grade, and I strongly recommend never using these products due to the risk of heavy-metal contamination.

If you believe that you can be helped by methylene blue, it's best to get a prescription for it and have it filled by a compounding pharmacist. This approach is far less expensive than using conventional pharmacies, which only sell it in 10 milliliter vials for IV use. These vials contain 100 milligrams and cost over $200.

My Current Methylene Blue Recommendations

I no longer take methylene blue regularly since I've found that daily walks in the ocean surf are an even better way to manage reductive stress. However, if I didn't have access to the ocean, I would likely take it six days a week. If you're considering it, I encourage you to speak with your doctor about whether it might be appropriate for your needs.

Most experts recommend relatively high doses for longer-term treatments of methylene blue, including dementia prevention and treatment, post-stroke care, cognitive enhancement, and overall health optimization. The doses they recommend are 0.5 milligram to 1 milligram per kilogram of body weight. For a person weighing 150 pounds, that would be a dose of 34–68 milligrams. I believe these doses are excessive and unnecessary. Doses of more than 3–5 milligrams are likely never needed unless you are undergoing treatment for some life-threatening conditions such as carbon monoxide or cyanide poisoning or a resistant urinary tract infection.

The average dose for most adults that reduces or eliminates reductive stress is only 5 milligrams, once a day, regardless of weight. It has a half-life of over twelve hours and will gradually build up if you take it every day, so higher doses are not needed. If you're using methylene blue to optimize the benefits of sun exposure, it's best to take it approximately thirty minutes before you plan to spend time in the sun.

Modulate Your Sun Exposure Based on How Long You Have Been Off Seed Oils

Dermatologists are right. Too much sun can prematurely age your skin and raise your cancer risk. But what they often don't emphasize is that it's not just the sun at play—it's also the vegetable oils in your diet. These oils accumulate in your skin and are then damaged by the sunlight, creating toxic compounds that can cause skin cancer and wrinkle your skin.

To truly protect your skin, consider the foods you eat as much as the time you spend in the sun. To reset your skin's health, make sure to eliminate vegetable oils and processed foods for at least six months before talking walks or sunbathing at solar noon. Over time, your body will rid itself of most of these harmful fats, allowing you to reap the sun's health benefits without the toxic side effects. During that interim period, avoid intense sun exposure during peak hours. Go out well before 10:00 a.m. or after 4:00 p.m. (for example, 9:00 a.m. or 7:00 p.m.). The sunlight isn't strong enough at those times to give you the exposure necessary for optimal health benefits, but it will keep you safe until the vegetable oils have been eliminated from your body.

Once you have decreased the toxic vegetable oils in your skin, then you can get your full dose of healthy sun exposure without added risk. At this point, shift to soaking up rays right around solar noon. That's about 12 noon, or 1 p.m. if it's daylight-saving time. Start with fifteen minutes or so and gradually build up the time you expose your skin to the sun.

This is the prime time to soak in the sun because the UV and near-infrared light are at their peak, which is what your body needs to energize itself and synthesize vitamin D. I walk at solar noon because I have been off vegetable oils for many years, so it's safe for me to do so.

You might be thinking, "But Dr. Mercola, I go for a walk every morning at 7:00 a.m. Isn't that good enough?" Well, I hate to break it to you, but not really, unless you are in your detoxing-from-vegetable-oil phase. If you take your walks too early in the morning or late in the evening, the sunlight isn't strong enough to give you the exposure you need for optimal health benefits.

Remember, proper sun exposure impacts nearly every aspect of your health. It's not just about avoiding vitamin D deficiency; it's about optimizing your entire biology. Sunlight at the right time can also regulate your sleep-wake cycle, boost your mood, and strengthen your immune system. It may also lower your risk of some cancers. It's nature's multivitamin, and it's free!

I've seen the difference proper sun exposure can make.

Tom, a friend of mine, told me about his low energy levels and frequent colds. He thought he was doing everything right—eating well, exercising, even taking vitamin D supplements. But when we dug deeper, we realized he was only getting sun exposure early in the morning. He adjusted his schedule to go outside at lunch, around noon. Within weeks, his energy soared, and he was sick less often.

So, here's my challenge to you: once you have detoxed vegetable oils, plan your day around a midday walk or outdoor break. Even fifteen to twenty minutes can make a substantial difference. If you work indoors, see if you can take your lunch outside or have walking meetings in the sunlight.

Rethinking Sunglasses: A New Perspective on Eye Health

Let's tackle a controversial topic: sunglasses. When you step out into a bright, sunny day, what's the first thing you do? Reach for your shades, right? Well, you might want to think twice about that habit. Your eyes, like the rest of your body, have evolved over millions of years to interact with sunlight. And just as your skin needs sunlight for vitamin D production, your eyes need natural light for optimal function.

When sunlight enters your eyes, it kicks off a whole cascade of beneficial processes in your body. It helps regulate your circadian rhythm, it affects your sleep and hormone production, and it even plays a role in preventing nearsightedness, especially in children. By habitually wearing sunglasses, you're inadvertently blocking these beneficial wavelengths of light. You're putting your eyes on a restrictive diet, depriving them of the full spectrum of light they need to function optimally.

Over time, constantly wearing sunglasses can lead to some unexpected problems. Your eyes might become more sensitive to light, making it uncomfortable to be outdoors without shades. Worse, it could cause myopia (nearsightedness), especially in developing children. Your brain relies on light exposure through your eyes to gauge the time of day and adjust your body's processes accordingly. Sunglasses send your brain confusing signals about the light, which can disrupt your natural rhythms.

I'm not saying you should never wear sunglasses. There are situations where it's advisable to limit excess light exposure. If you're skiing on a sunny day, wear those shades. The snow-covered slopes will reflect light from all directions. If you're by the open ocean, the sun will glare off the water's surface. In these extreme conditions, the amount of light reaching your eyes can be overwhelming and harmful to them.

The key is balance and context. Before grabbing your sunglasses, consider the outdoors and how long you'll be outside. For everyday activities, try to embrace natural light. Let your eyes adapt to the brightness gradually. You might be surprised at how quickly your eyes adjust and how much more vibrant and alive the world appears without the filter of sunglasses.

Vitamin D: The Sunshine Vitamin

When you step outside on a sunny day, something amazing happens. The sun's ultraviolet B (UVB) rays hit your skin, kicking off a chain reaction that produces vitamin D. It's as if your body has a little vitamin factory and sunlight is the on switch. But vitamin D isn't just about strong bones—it's a powerhouse nutrient that affects nearly every aspect of your health.

Let's start with the basics. Yes, vitamin D helps your body absorb calcium, which is crucial for building and maintaining strong bones. Without enough vitamin D, you're at risk for conditions like osteoporosis, where your bones become weak and brittle. But vitamin D does a whole lot more than that. It acts as a master regulator in your body, influencing over 2,500 genes. It's akin to a conductor directing a massive orchestra of biological processes.

This vitamin plays a role in preventing and fighting several serious diseases. Vitamin D has been linked to lower risks of some cancers, type 2 diabetes, and respiratory infections. It may even lower the risk of autoimmune diseases like multiple sclerosis.

How does vitamin D do it all? One way is by modulating your immune system. Vitamin D boosts your innate immune system—your body's first line of defense—by increasing the production of antimicrobial peptides. These are like your body's own natural antibiotics. It also helps manage the behavior of T and B cells in your adaptive immune system, which is responsible for creating a targeted response to specific threats.

Vitamin D is also a powerful anti-inflammatory agent, helping to keep chronic inflammation in check. This is crucial because chronic inflammation is at the root of many modern diseases, including heart disease and cancer. Vitamin D is also essential for proper cell growth and differentiation, which ensures that your body's cells are developing and functioning as they should.

When it comes to physical performance and recovery, vitamin D is again a key player. It supports muscle function and helps your body recover from injury or intense exercise. It even plays a role in lung function, which is pivotal for athletes and anyone dealing with respiratory issues. And let's not forget about mental health—vitamin D has been linked to lower rates of depression and anxiety. It's a mood booster that comes straight from the sun.

Vitamin D: Your Body's Energy Regulator
The way vitamin D helps regulate your body's energy production comes down to its interaction with an enzyme called AMP-activated protein kinase, or AMPK. Think of AMPK as your body's metabolic master switch. It's constantly monitoring the energy status of your cells, and when energy levels drop, it springs into action.

Here's how it works: AMPK is sensitive to the ratio of AMP (adenosine monophosphate) to ATP (adenosine triphosphate) in your cells. ATP is your body's main energy currency, and when it's used up, it's converted to AMP. When AMPK detects a high AMP-to-ATP ratio, it raises a red flag signaling that your cells' energy reserves are running low. In response, AMPK kicks off processes to generate more ATP and puts a temporary halt on energy-consuming processes.

This is where vitamin D comes in. It plays an instrumental role in supporting AMPK activation, which has a whole host of benefits. First, AMPK increases the efficiency of ATP production. This is necessary for high-energy tissues like your muscles and brain. When AMPK is active, it also enhances glucose uptake into your cells, aiding them in producing more energy. This helps maintain healthy blood sugar levels, which can be a game-changer for those with insulin resistance or type 2 diabetes.

AMPK activation also encourages fat burning, which helps with weight management and reduces the risk of obesity-related diseases. It also has strong anti-inflammatory effects.

One of the most fascinating aspects of AMPK activation is its role in autophagy. This is your cells' self-cleaning process, clearing out damaged parts and helping the cells rejuvenate themselves. This is essential for preventing diseases and promoting longevity. Keeping your vitamin D levels optimal ensures that AMPK works efficiently, which will regulate your energy balance, boost your metabolism, and protect against diseases.

Vitamin D: Your Antiaging Ally

Vitamin D even plays a significant role in how you age. Recent studies have shed light on just how fundamental this nutrient is in the aging process. A groundbreaking study published in 2024 highlighted the impact of vitamin D on twelve key aging markers. Those affected include genomic instability, changes in gene expression, and issues with protein function.

The researchers also looked at how vitamin D impacts the following:

- Cellular recycling efficiency
- Nutrient-sensing disruptions
- Mitochondrial problems
- Cell aging
- Stem cell depletion
- Chronic inflammation
- Gut flora imbalance

All these markers are interconnected and contribute to the cellular and molecular damage we see as we age. The exciting part is that vitamin D helps mitigate this damage. It's particularly beneficial for mitochondrial function and helps reduce oxidative stress, a major player in aging.

Another fascinating aspect of vitamin D's antiaging effects is its influence on DNA methylation. This is a process where DNA activity is regulated by adding methyl groups to the DNA molecule, affecting which genes are turned on or off. The length of these groups is a common measure of biological aging, but epigenetic clocks, which look at DNA methylation patterns, are more accurate. Vitamin D helps regulate methylation, which keeps your biological age lower.

The study also explored whether vitamin D could curb cellular aging. It aimed to reduce the senescence-associated secretory phenotype (SASP). In simpler terms, vitamin D might help stop older cells from releasing inflammatory molecules that can damage nearby healthy cells. By supplementing with vitamin D, we might be able to reduce these harmful effects and slow down the aging process at a cellular level.

We can see that getting enough vitamin D could be a low-cost way to feel younger. It also helps keep your body's cells working their best.

Vitamin D: Your Body's Natural Cancer Fighter
You might not know it, but vitamin D can also be a powerful weapon in your body's fight against cancer. Cancer is marked by uncontrolled cell growth, and vitamin D is an important part of regulating cell growth. Vitamin D interacts with something called the vitamin D receptor (VDR) in your cells. When vitamin D binds to this receptor, it triggers a series of biochemical signals that tell your cells how to behave properly. This includes their growth, development, and survival.

Vitamin D also activates pathways involving molecules like Nrf2. This defends the cells against oxidative stress and DNA damage that can lead to cancer.

The research on vitamin D and cancer is mind-blowing. Studies show that a vitamin D level of at least 40 ng/mL could reduce your cancer risk by 67 percent. This is compared to having levels of 20 ng/mL or less. That's a substantial difference! And it's not just about prevention. Higher vitamin D levels may improve outcomes in breast, colorectal, lung, prostate, bladder, and other cancers.

Sunlight: Nature's Melatonin Booster

Here's another amazing way sunlight helps your body: by boosting melatonin production. You probably know melatonin as the "sleep hormone," but there's a lot more to it than that. Sunlight exposure causes near-infrared rays to penetrate your skin and reach your mito-chondria. This stimulates the production of melatonin right there in the mitochondria.

In fact, 95 percent of the melatonin in your body is produced in your mitochondria, not in your brain, as previously thought. This mitochondrial melatonin is different from the melatonin in your pineal gland that helps regulate your sleep-wake cycle. Instead, mitochondrial melatonin acts as a powerful antioxidant, neutralizing harmful ROS. These ROS can damage your cells and DNA, leading to inflammation and various chronic diseases, including cancer.

But the benefits of this sunlight-induced melatonin production don't stop there. An additional full range of health advantages include:

- Protecting your heart by reducing oxidative stress, inflamma-tion, and cell death

- Shielding your kidneys from damage by reducing oxidative stress and inflammation

- Activating powerful anti-inflammatory responses throughout your body

- Enhancing your body's natural antioxidant defenses

- Helping to prevent cancer by protecting against cellular damage

- Supporting metabolic health by regulating insulin signaling and mitochondrial function

- Protecting your brain from oxidative stress and inflammation, potentially helping prevent neurodegenerative diseases

- Modulating your immune response, helping to protect against infections and autoimmune diseases

Even though the morning sun isn't strong enough to trigger vita-min D production, it plays a powerful role in resetting your body's master clock. This master clock, in your brain's suprachiasmatic nucleus (SCN), is like an orchestra's conductor. It ensures all the little clocks in your body work together in harmony.

When morning light enters your eyes and reaches the SCN, it's like a wake-up call for your entire body. It tells your brain, "Hey, it's daytime now!" and prompts the SCN to reset itself to match the new day. This reset is necessary to regulate your sleep-wake cycle, synchronizing your body's clock with the outside world.

Moreover, recent research found another link between vitamin D and your circadian system. Scientists have discovered that blood vitamin D levels change throughout the day. They also follow a circadian rhythm. They've even found that vitamin D influences the activity of circadian genes in fat-tissue cells.

Even more intriguing is that a protein called Clock, which is crucial for our circadian rhythm, interacts with the vitamin D receptor. This interaction helps the vitamin D receptor bind to its target DNA, suggesting a close relationship between vitamin D and our internal clock.

Lastly, vitamin D is believed to play a role in regulating the sleep-wake cycle itself. Studies have found that low levels of vitamin D are linked to poor sleep quality and shorter sleep duration. Some researchers have proposed a direct link between sleep disorders and low vitamin D levels in the body.

This is why I always recommend getting some morning sunlight exposure, in addition to midday sun for vitamin D production. It is a simple, natural way to keep your body's clocks running smoothly. This can lead to enhanced quality of sleep, improved mood, better digestion, and superior overall health.

Improve Your Mental Health and Sleep Quality with Sunlight

If you've ever felt a lift in your spirits on a sunny day, there's a scientific reason for that. Sunlight exposure triggers the production of endorphins in your body. These are the same chemicals that give you a "runner's high," acting as natural painkillers and mood elevators. Sunshine boosts your endorphin levels, improving your mood and reducing stress and anxiety.

This mood-boosting effect of sunlight is key for those with Seasonal Affective Disorder (SAD). SAD is a type of seasonal depression that starts in the fall and lasts through winter, when the days are shorter. It's not just a case of the "winter blues." It can be a serious condition that significantly affects quality of life. The good news is that bright-light therapy, which mimics natural sunlight, is a well-recognized and effective treatment for SAD.

Proper sunlight exposure is also linked to better sleep quality, which in turn is essential for good mental health. Poor sleep is often associated with higher levels of depression and anxiety. Sunlight exposure can regulate your circadian rhythms—your body's internal clock so that you are able to attain better sleep. And better sleep leads to better mental health.

The ideal way to get vitamin D is through sun exposure on bare skin. This is because your skin is an incredible organ, capable of producing up to 25,000 international units (IU) of vitamin D on a sunny day. That's a staggering amount, especially when you consider that many vitamin D supplements contain only 1,000 to 2,000 IU per dose.

Despite this, most people aren't getting enough sun to maintain optimal vitamin D levels. Our indoor, modern lives are missing out on a free, healthy source of this essential vitamin. And it's not just a problem in colder, darker climates. Even in sunny areas, people who stay indoors or use sunscreen often have low vitamin D.

You might have heard that a vitamin D level of 20 ng/mL is the cutoff for deficiency. But I'm here to tell you that this number is far too low for truly vibrant health and disease prevention. If you want to give your body the vitamin D it needs to thrive and protect itself against illnesses like cancer, you should be aiming higher. The sweet spot for vitamin D is between 60 ng/mL and 80 ng/mL (150-200 nmol/L). This is the range where your body can really work its magic, optimizing your health and fortifying your defenses against disease.

The Smart Way to Check for Sun Overexposure Is with the Sunburn Test

Even though sun exposure is the ideal way to get vitamin D, it is a double-edged sword. Sun exposure has a complex interplay of benefits and risks, deeply influenced by your diet, environment, and physiology. While it's essential for vitamin D production and health, it can also be harmful if you're not careful. The key is understanding how to protect yourself while still reaping the benefits. Let's talk about some strategies that can help you achieve that balance.

As mentioned earlier, if you've been eating a diet high in vegetable oils or seed oils, you need to be extra cautious with sun exposure. These oils are rich in linoleic acid (LA), an omega-6 fat that is highly prone to oxidation when exposed to UV radiation. When sunlight interacts with skin containing these oils, it causes the oils to break down, leading to inflammation and DNA damage. That's why I recommend avoiding sun exposure unless you've eliminated seed oils from your diet for at least six months.

The relationship between sun exposure and your health is further modulated by your environment and physical characteristics. For example, higher elevations have thinner atmospheres, allowing more UVB rays—the type responsible for vitamin D production—to reach the Earth's surface. This explains why sun exposure at high altitudes can be more potent, both in terms of benefits and risks.

Similarly, atmospheric conditions such as cloud cover and air pollution play a role. Thick clouds or smog can block UVB rays, reducing both vitamin D production and the risk of sunburn. This variability in UV penetration highlights the need for awareness of our local environment when planning sun exposure.

Individual physical characteristics also influence your relationship with the sun. Skin color, determined by melanin content, is a prime example. Melanin acts as a natural sunscreen, meaning darker-skinned individuals require more sun exposure to produce the same amount of vitamin D as those with lighter skin. This biological variation emphasizes the need for personalized approaches to sun exposure.

Body composition, particularly fat percentage, is another determining factor. Adipose tissue can store fat-soluble compounds, including oxidized vegetable oils. Individuals with higher body fat percentages may therefore need to be more cautious, as these stored oils can prolong the risk period even after dietary changes.

Geographical location and seasonal variations add another layer of complexity. Areas with long winters and overcast weather naturally limit sun exposure, reducing both benefits and risks. Winter clothing also minimizes sun exposure. So, even if you are still consuming seed oils, there is minimal risk to your health in the winter, as the oils are not being oxidized by UV radiation.

The best way to assess your sun exposure, especially if you have a history of consuming vegetable oils, is to monitor your skin for any signs of redness or burning. This simple "sunburn test" considers all the variables discussed above—physical characteristics, geographical locations, and seasonal variations. If you don't notice even the slightest hint of pink on your skin, it's a good sign that your sun exposure was within a safe range. Always aim to avoid sunburn, as it indicates overexposure.

You might be wondering, "Dr. Mercola, what if I've already reduced my intake of these oils?" Well, that's great news! As you lower your body's stores of LA, your risk of sunburn and skin cancer decreases dramatically. However, it's still important to be mindful of your sun exposure, especially during the transition period.

As you begin reducing vegetable and seed oils in your diet, avoid peak sunlight hours, which are typically an hour before and after solar noon. In most of the US during summer, this means staying out of direct sun from 11:00 a.m. to 3:00 p.m. during daylight saving time, or 10:00 a.m. to 2:00 p.m. in standard time. Eventually, as your body detoxes the accumulated vegetable and seed oils, you can gradually increase your time in the sun. Ultimately, you will be able to enjoy an hour or more of peak sunlight hours.

Remember, everyone's skin is different, so listen to your body during this adjustment period. The key is to never let your skin burn. Sunburn is a sign of damage—if you notice any redness, seek shade at once. By being mindful of your sun exposure, you're taking an important step in caring for your health. So, pay close attention to your skin. It's your body's way of communicating with you. Again, UV rays will interact with vegetable oils embedded in your skin cells, increasing your risk of wrinkles on your face, sunburn and, over time, skin cancer.

If you do need to spend time in the sun before your body has fully cleared out these oils, there are some protective strategies you can implement. One of my favorite recommendations is astaxanthin, a powerful antioxidant found in certain marine life. Taking 12 milligrams of astaxanthin once a day can help increase your skin's resistance to sun damage. It works by neutralizing free radicals and reducing inflammation. This gives your skin extra protection against UV radiation.

Another helpful tool in your sun-protection arsenal is niacinamide cream. Niacinamide, also known as vitamin B3, has been shown to help protect against UV-induced DNA damage when applied topically. It can also improve your skin's barrier, making it more resilient to stressors like sun exposure. I've seen patients have remarkable success with applying niacinamide cream before sun exposure.

Here's a tip that might surprise you. Taking a baby aspirin thirty to sixty minutes before sun exposure could lower your risk of skin cancer. Aspirin prevents the LA in your skin from turning into harmful OXLAMs (oxidized linoleic acid metabolites). These OXLAMs are a primary contributor not just to skin cancer but to many types of cancer. By inhibiting their formation, aspirin can provide an extra layer of protection against sun damage.

Molecular hydrogen (H_2) offers another layer of protection against sun damage and mitigates the harmful effects of vegetable oils. This remarkable molecule works at the cellular level, effectively reducing oxidative stress by neutralizing harmful free radicals, with a particular affinity for the highly reactive hydroxyl radical.

H_2's unique properties allow it to penetrate cell membranes easily, directly targeting sources of inflammation and oxidative damage. Importantly, it does this without interfering with beneficial ROS, maintaining the body's delicate oxidative balance.

Beyond this protective role, molecular hydrogen also provides other benefits, including increased energy levels and enhanced exercise recovery. This makes H_2 a valuable tool in your arsenal for supporting cellular health, especially when facing environmental stressors like sun exposure or dietary challenges from vegetable oil consumption.

Building Natural Sun Resilience: A Holistic Approach to Healthier Sun Exposure

It's important to note that these strategies are not a substitute for sensible sun exposure. They're tools to help protect you while you're transitioning to a healthier diet and lifestyle. The goal is to get your body to a point where it can handle reasonable sun exposure without relying on these extra protections.

In my medical career, I've seen remarkable transformations in people who have followed this approach. Sarah is a friend of mine who has a history of frequent sunburns and a family history of skin cancer. She was understandably nervous about sun exposure. We worked together to adjust her diet, eliminate seed oils, and implement the protective strategies I've discussed.

After about eight months, Sarah was amazed to find that she could spend time in the sun without burning. Her skin had become more resilient, and she was able to enjoy outdoor activities without constant fear of sun damage.

Another friend, John, was an avid cyclist who spent hours in the sun every week. Despite using high-SPF sunscreens, he often ended up with sunburn and was worried about his long-term skin health. We implemented a similar protocol, focusing on dietary changes and targeted supplements. Within a year, John reported that he no longer needed to rely on chemical sunscreens. His skin had grown more resilient to the sun. Now, he can enjoy cycling without harming his skin.

These success stories highlight an important point. Your skin's reaction to the sun reflects your internal health. If you address the root causes of sun sensitivity, you will greatly improve your skin's resilience to the sun. Remember, the goal isn't to avoid the sun entirely. The key is to increase your body's natural resilience so that you can safely enjoy the benefits of sunlight without excessive risk of damage to your skin.

As you put these strategies in place, pay close attention to how your skin responds to sun exposure. Over time, you should notice that you're able to spend more time in the sun without burning. This is a sign that your body is becoming more efficient at handling UV radiation. But always err on the side of caution and avoid overexposure, especially during peak sunlight hours and the hottest parts of the day.

Structured Sun Exposure: Maximizing Benefits, Minimizing Risks
We've established that moderate sun exposure has a myriad of health benefits, but some of you may still be asking, "Dr. Mercola, what about skin cancer?" Here's the truth the mainstream medical establishment won't tell you: melanoma, the most serious skin cancer, isn't necessarily caused by direct sun exposure.

It's well-recognized that many skin cancers develop in areas of the body that rarely or never see the light of day. What's more, we've already discussed how vitamin D, the very thing your skin produces when exposed to sunlight, is a powerful anticancer agent. It cuts your risk of developing over a dozen deadly cancers, which are more common than melanoma.

The melanin in your skin is another part of your skin's built-in cancer protection. This is the pigment that darkens your skin in the sun. It acts like a natural sunscreen, absorbing UV rays and protecting your skin cells from DNA damage. Interestingly, melanin production is activated by the release of beta-endorphins in response to sunlight. So not only are you protecting your skin, but you're also getting a little mood boost in the process!

The key to safe sun exposure is to build up your tan gradually. Start by exposing substantial portions of skin for only five to fifteen minutes at a time if you're fair-skinned, and longer if you have naturally darker skin. You want your skin to develop just the slightest hint of pink, then cover back up. Each day after that, add a few more minutes. This allows your melanin to do its job and protect your skin cells from UV damage. If you start this process in the spring, by midsummer you'll be able to spend hours outside without burning, and your risk of skin cancer will be minimal.

Embracing the Sun's Power: A Path to Optimal Health

Let's recap the key points we've covered. We examined the sun's role as the source of energy for all life on Earth. Then, we explored the world of electrons. They transfer energy from the sun to every cell in your body. We then reviewed the health benefits of sun exposure. It boosts vitamin D and positively affects heart and immune health.

We've debunked the myth that sun exposure is harmful. Studies show that moderate sun exposure is linked to lower mortality and better health. We've explored sunlight as an unrecognized nutrient. We drew parallels between human health and plant growth that show the impact of adequate sun exposure on your overall well-being.

Our journey took us into cellular energy production, which introduced the groundbreaking concept of photometabolism. We've explored how our bodies can harness energy directly from the sun. We've talked about the risks of energy production, like reductive stress. We've explored natural solutions, like grounding and methylene blue, to boost our energy systems.

We've given practical advice on how to maximize sun exposure. We emphasized the importance of timing. We explained why midday sun is best for vitamin D and health and even challenged the old view on eye protection.

Throughout this exploration, a central theme has emerged: the sun is not our enemy, but a vital ally in our quest for optimal health. By working with your body's natural processes, you can harness the power of sunlight. It can boost your energy, mood, and overall well-being. The key is finding the right balance. Get enough sun to enjoy its benefits. But be careful of skin damage from too much exposure.

As you move forward, I encourage you to view sunlight in a new light (pun intended). Embrace it as an essential nutrient, a free and abundant resource that your body is designed to use for optimal function. Try to get some midday sun every day and add mindful sun exposure to your daily routine. Pay attention to how your body feels and responds as you make these changes.

Remember, your health journey is unique to you. What works for one person may need to be altered for another. Listen to your body. Be patient with the process. Seek guidance from a health-care professional who values natural health. Respecting and working with nature's rhythms, including the sun's daily cycle, is a powerful step toward vibrant and lasting good health.

Your Path to Vibrant Health Begins with a Single Step: Discover the Joy of Movement

Your ancestors didn't need a gym membership to stay fit. They were in constant motion, walking miles to gather food, sprinting to hunt prey, and climbing trees to harvest fruit. This wasn't just about survival; it was the key to their vibrant health. Fast forward to today, and you might see people spending hours hunched over a desk, slouched on a couch, or stuck in traffic. This sedentary lifestyle is a far cry from what your body was designed for, and it's taking a toll on your health in ways you might not even realize.

When you move, magic happens inside your body. Blood starts pumping faster, delivering a surge of oxygen and nutrients to every cell. Your lymphatic system kicks into high gear, flushing out toxins and boosting your immune function. Even your brain gets a boost. With each step you take, a cascade of chemicals is released into your system—lifting your mood and sharpening your mind. It's like giving your body a tune-up from the inside out.

Think about how you feel after sitting for hours. Stiff, sluggish, maybe even a bit foggy. That's your body sending you an SOS signal.

It's crying out for movement. Just as a lack of sunlight can leave you deficient in vitamin D, a lack of movement starves your body of the physical stimulation it craves. The result of a sedentary lifestyle is that a host of health problems can creep up on you, from heart disease to depression.

But the good news is you don't need to become a marathon runner to reap the benefits of movement. The key is to weave physical activity back into the fabric of your daily life. Stand up while you're on the phone, take the stairs instead of the elevator, or have a walking meeting instead of sitting in a conference room. These small changes can easily add up to big health benefits over time.

Take Control of Your Health: The Power of Moving More Every Day

Here's what happens to your body when you don't move enough. First, your metabolic rate takes a nosedive. Think of your metabolism as your body's engine. When you're active, it revs up, burning calories efficiently. When you're sedentary, it slows to a crawl. This doesn't just make it harder to maintain a healthy weight, it throws off the balance of your whole energy-producing system.

But that's just the beginning. Your muscles, those powerhouses of movement and metabolism, start to waste away in a process called atrophy. Over time, this can lead to sarcopenia, a fancy term for age-related muscle loss. You might think, "So what if I lose a little muscle?" You might not realize it, but your muscles are metabolically active even when you're at rest. This means when you lose muscle mass, whether you are in motion or not, you're essentially downgrading your body's calorie-burning engine.

Then there's the issue of insulin sensitivity. When you're inactive, your muscles use less glucose and need less insulin to absorb it. Over time, this reduced demand for insulin can cause your body to become less responsive to it, leading to insulin resistance. This is a slippery slope that can end in type 2 diabetes, with all its nasty side effects—nerve damage, kidney disease, and vision problems.

Your heart, that tireless muscle pumping away in your chest, doesn't escape the effects of inactivity either. Just like any other muscle, it needs regular exercise to stay strong. When you're sedentary, your heart can weaken, becoming less effective at its job. This can eventually lead to many cardiovascular problems, including heart failure. And let's not forget about blood pressure. A lack of physical activity can cause it to creep up, putting extra strain on your heart and blood vessels.

And it's not just adults who need to worry about this. A recent study found that kids who are too sedentary are at risk for heart problems later in life. Those with too little moderate-to-vigorous activity are more likely to have a higher cardiac workload and more body fat—both risk factors for heart disease.

You might say, "But I hit the gym a few times a week. Isn't that enough?" Unfortunately, research shows that even if you exercise regularly, prolonged periods of sitting can still harm your health. One study found that six hours of uninterrupted sitting effectively cancels out the benefits of a full hour of exercise.

So, what's the solution? It's simple: attempt to move more throughout your entire day. Stand up every hour, take short walks, do some stretches. Your body will thank you for it. Remember, the human body is designed for movement. When you deny that basic need, you're inviting a whole host of health problems.

I've seen countless patients improve their health by simply moving more. One patient, let's call her Sarah, came to me complaining of chronic fatigue, weight gain, and mood swings. She had a demanding office job that kept her chained to her desk for hours on end. We started small, with hourly movement breaks and a standing desk. Within weeks, she reported feeling more energetic. Her mood had improved, and she even began to lose weight without changing her diet.

Derek, another patient, was prediabetic and struggling with high blood pressure. He was resistant to the idea of exercise, associating it with grueling gym sessions. We focused on adding more natural movement to his day. For example, he started parking farther from store entrances, taking his dog for longer walks, and doing calf raises while brushing his teeth. Six months later, his blood sugar levels had normalized, and his blood pressure was back in a healthy range.

These stories aren't unique. They're powerful examples of what can happen when you give your body the movement it craves. It's not about punishing yourself with intense workouts (unless that's what you enjoy). It's about returning to a more natural state of frequent, varied movement throughout your day.

Think about it: every time you stand up, take a walk, or climb a flight of stairs, you're giving your body a mini tune-up. You're boosting your metabolism, strengthening your heart, and improving your insulin sensitivity. You're also giving your brain a little workout. It's like making a series of small deposits into your health bank account. Over time, these deposits add up to significant gains in your well-being.

So, I challenge you to take a hard look at your daily routine. How much time do you spend sitting? How can you incorporate more movement into your day? Could you do some bodyweight exercises during TV commercial breaks? Could you set a timer to remind you to move every hour?

Your body is an amazing machine designed for movement. When you honor that design, you're paving the way for better health, more energy, and a higher quality of life. It's time to get moving, not just for your physical health, but for your mental and emotional health as well.

The Hidden Dangers of a Slow Metabolism

You've heard people blame their weight problems on a "slow metabolism." But a slow metabolic rate affects more than just your waistline. It's as if your body's transmission is stuck in first gear—it impacts every aspect of your health and well-being. Let's examine the consequences of a sluggish metabolism and how you can rev it up.

When your metabolism slows down, weight gain is often the first noticeable sign. Your body becomes less efficient at burning calories, so any excess calories are stored as fat. This isn't just about fitting into your favorite jeans; carrying extra weight puts a serious strain on your heart and blood vessels. It's a recipe for high blood pressure, hardened arteries, and an increased risk of heart attacks and strokes. Think of it as your body's pipes getting clogged and overworked.

A slow metabolism can also cause insulin resistance. When this happens, your cells become less responsive to insulin and its management of your blood sugar. As a result, glucose builds up in your bloodstream, setting the stage for type 2 diabetes and its numerous related health problems.

Sometimes, a sluggish metabolism is a sign of an underactive thyroid gland. Your thyroid is like the thermostat for your body's energy production. When it's not producing enough hormones, everything slows down. You might feel constantly tired, gain weight easily, and even experience depression.

A slow metabolism can take a serious toll on your mood and cognitive function too. When you don't have enough energy, you might feel chronically fatigued, unmotivated, or even depressed. It's hard to concentrate or remember things, which affects your work and relationships. Here's a mind-blowing fact: your brain only makes up 2 percent of your body weight, but it uses 20 percent of your energy. So, when your metabolism is low, your brain is one of the first things to feel the effects.

Perhaps most frustratingly, a slow metabolism can leave you feeling like you are stuck in a rut. Changing your life takes a lot of cellular energy. Having a slow metabolism makes implementing changes—including starting a new hobby, switching careers, or improving relationships—even more of a daunting challenge. When your metabolism is slow, that energy just isn't there. It's like trying to run a marathon on an empty tank.

How Measuring Your Body Temperature Helps You Master Your Metabolism

How do you determine if your metabolism is running hot or cold? Think of your body as a furnace, constantly burning fuel to keep you warm and energized. The hotter that furnace runs, the more efficiently your body is working. One of the easiest ways to gauge the heat of your metabolic fire is by measuring your body temperature.

When your body temperature is low, your internal furnace is running on low heat. You might have cold hands and feet, thinning hair, and digestive issues. You may feel very tired. These are all signs that your metabolic fire needs stoking. Your furnace needs a jump start.

Conversely, when your metabolism is running hot, you reap a host of benefits. You can eat more without gaining weight. You have more energy, better body composition, and improved digestion and detox. You can enjoy a wider variety of foods, sleep better, and generally feel better, like you're living life to the fullest. It's similar to upgrading from an old clunker to a high-performance sports car.

Measuring your metabolic rate is as simple as taking your temperature throughout the day, starting from the moment you wake up. The higher your body temperature, the more heat—and therefore energy—your body is producing. Ideally, your waking temperature should be in the high 97s to low 98s Fahrenheit. After breakfast, your body temperature should rise. It should peak at 98.6°F by midday or early afternoon. Then, it should slowly decline as bedtime approaches.

One thing to note: stress hormones can raise your morning temperature. Make sure to take many readings throughout the day. This will help find any metabolic slowdown. Once you've eaten breakfast and those stress hormone levels normalize, you'll get a truer picture of your metabolic health. If your morning temps are high but drop after eating, it's a red flag. Your thyroid and metabolism are sluggish and propped up by stress hormones. A truly metabolism-boosting meal should increase both body heat and energy production.

Keeping your body temperature high is also necessary for optimal organ function. Your enzymes, the biological machines that keep your body running, work best at specific temperatures. Even a small drop in body temp can harm enzyme activity. It can weaken your immune system, making you more vulnerable to disease. Dr. Hiromi Shinya at the Albert Einstein College of Medicine found that a 0.9°F drop in body temperature can reduce enzyme and immune activity by 30 percent. He also found that cancer cells multiply much faster at 95°F than at 98.6°F.

Alarmingly, low body temperatures are becoming increasingly common, though they're far from normal. The average body temperature used to be a steady 98.6°F, but it's been dropping as obesity rates have climbed. Environmental toxins, hormone-disrupting chemicals, and undernourishment are causing this decline. So are low-carb diets, chronic stress, and diets high in polyunsaturated fatty acids (PUFAs).

If your temperature readings are consistently low, consider it a wake-up call to make some changes and rev up your metabolism:

- Eat enough calories.

- Cut back on PUFAs.

- Choose carbs that suit your body.

- Do strength training.

- Manage stress.

- Make time for Joy and creativity.

- Avoid extreme diets, like prolonged fasting or very low-carb eating. They can harm your metabolism in the long run.

Taking your pulse alongside your temperature can provide even more insight into your metabolic health. Your pulse shows how efficiently nutrients and energy are reaching your cells. High temperatures and low pulse rates are strong indications that you have a slow metabolism. Aim to stay in the 70 to 90/95 BPM (beats per minute) range for optimal health. Contrary to popular belief, a low heart rate isn't always a good thing. While it may help athletes perform better in the short term, over time it can speed up aging, dampen libido, and hinder digestion.

By tracking your body temperature and adjusting your lifestyle, you can boost your metabolism. As your temperature rises, your symptoms will fade. Your energy and health will soar. Your metabolic fire will be burning hot, and you'll be ready to take on the world. A healthy metabolism is more than just weight management. It's the key to your body's full potential for vitality and well-being.

Powering Up Your Cellular Engines

When you exercise, you're doing much more than just burning calories or building muscle. You're giving your cells a complete overhaul. This includes the tiny powerhouses within them, the mitochondria. These microscopic energy factories are key to your vitality—physical activity is a turbo boost for their function and production.

Let's talk about mitochondrial biogenesis—a medical term for your body's ability to create new mitochondria. When you engage in regular physical activity, you're sending a powerful signal to your cells that they need to step up their game. It's like telling your body,

"Hey, we need more energy around here!" In response, your cells start churning out new mitochondria to meet the increased demand.

The key orchestrator in this process is a molecule called PGC-1α. Envision PGC-1α as a master gardener in a vast cellular greenhouse. When you exercise, PGC-1α springs into action, sowing seeds and nurturing a diverse array of genes involved in energy metabolism. It's like activating an advanced irrigation system, providing the perfect amount of nutrients and care to stimulate rapid growth of mitochondrial "plants" throughout your cellular garden.

The importance of increasing mitochondrial numbers cannot be overstated. Picture transforming a small, local power plant into a sprawling, state-of-the-art energy grid. That's essentially what you're doing for your body at a cellular level. With more mitochondria, your cells can convert nutrients into usable energy (ATP) much more efficiently. This means your body can operate at peak performance, handling increased energy demands with ease and resilience.

But the benefits don't stop there. These extra mitochondria keep working even when you're at rest, ensuring your cells always have the energy they need. It's like having a team of tireless workers constantly ready to meet your body's energy demands. This efficiency boosts your health. It gives you stable energy and more endurance for all your activities.

There's another key benefit of mitochondrial biogenesis that's often overlooked—better waste management in cells. Your mitochondria aren't just energy producers; they're also your cells' cleanup crew. When they work well, they help dispose of toxic byproducts. These can accumulate and cause oxidative stress when they are not removed effectively. Exercise boosts your mitochondria, making them more efficient, upgrading your body's waste disposal system, and keeping your cells cleaner and healthier.

I've seen the transformative power of mitochondrial enhancement firsthand. One patient, let's call him Tom, came to me complaining of chronic fatigue and weight gain despite a seemingly healthy diet. We implemented a regular exercise routine focusing on both aerobic and resistance training. Within weeks, Tom reported a noticeable increase in his energy levels. After a few months, not only had he lost weight, but he also found he needed less sleep and recovered faster from his workouts. This is the power of optimized mitochondrial function in action.

Exercise Is Your Key to Unlocking Unlimited Energy to Prevent Disease

We've discussed how lack of exercise or a slow metabolism can lead to insulin resistance. Now, let's explore how exercise can reverse this trend. Imagine your body as a vast postal system. Insulin acts as the central sorting office, responsible for directing packages of glucose—your body's primary fuel—to various destinations (your cells) across the network. In this scenario, exercise functions like an efficiency expert brought in to overhaul the entire operation.

When you exercise regularly, the efficiency expert is implementing a series of improvements throughout the system. They're streamlining processes, upgrading equipment, and training staff to handle packages more effectively. As a result, packages (glucose) are delivered more quickly and accurately to their intended recipients (cells), with less need for oversight from the central sorting office (insulin).

Over time, these improvements lead to a more responsive, efficient delivery system that requires less intervention from the central sorting office to maintain smooth operations. This enhanced capability is what we call increased insulin sensitivity. The system becomes so well-tuned that it can handle its workload with minimal strain. A fit body can process glucose more effectively with less insulin. As a result of this increased systemwide efficiency, your body will use glucose more efficiently even during recovery and rest.

But wait, there's more! Exercise also helps reduce inflammatory markers in your body. These inflammatory substances are roadblocks that contribute to the chaos in your body caused by insulin resistance. Exercise keeps the roads clear for insulin and glucose, which improves insulin sensitivity.

Overall, exercise builds a strong defense against many diseases. Take type 2 diabetes, for example. This metabolic disorder is rampant. The good news is, it can often be managed or even prevented through regular exercise. By making your body more responsive to insulin, exercise helps keep your blood sugar levels in check. This may mean you need less medication. It also lowers your risk of health issues like nerve damage, vision problems, and heart disease.

Better insulin sensitivity protects you from metabolic syndrome, which is a dangerous mix of high blood pressure, high blood sugar, excess belly fat, and bad cholesterol. When these conditions gang up, they significantly increase your risk of heart disease, stroke, and type 2 diabetes. But exercising regularly can reduce your disease risk by tackling many aspects of metabolic syndrome head-on.

I once worked with a patient, Mary, who was on the brink of being diagnosed with type 2 diabetes. Her blood sugar levels were consistently high, and her doctor was ready to start her on medication. Instead, we implemented a comprehensive exercise program, combining resistance training with daily walks. Within three months, Mary's blood sugar levels had normalized, and she had lost fifteen pounds. More importantly, for the first time in years, she felt energized and in control of her health.

So, when you exercise, you're not just burning calories. You're also optimizing your body's energy delivery system. You're training your muscles to absorb glucose better, lowering your body's insulin demand and, in general, creating a healthier metabolic environment.

The beauty of exercise is that unlike many medications, which have many potential adverse effects, exercise has none; it's part of a holistic approach to health that addresses many aspects of your physiology at once.

If you have health issues or want to boost your well-being, exercise is key. It's one of the best steps you can take. Just start where you are—a daily walk, a few minutes of bodyweight exercises, or a bike ride around the neighborhood. The key is consistency and gradual progression. Your body is wonderfully adaptive, and with time and persistence, you'll be amazed at the positive changes you'll see and feel.

Harmonize Your Hormones and Revitalize Your Body with Every Move

You might think of exercise primarily as a way to build muscle or lose weight, but it's time to expand your perspective. When you move, you're not just burning calories. You're also fine-tuning your endocrine system.

Let's talk about how exercise functions as a hormone balancer. Physical activity sends signals throughout your body that affect hormone production and regulation. It's like flipping a series of switches, with each one affecting a different aspect of your physiology. This hormonal dance impacts everything from your mood and energy levels to your metabolism and sleep patterns.

One interesting effect of exercise on hormones is its impact on estrogen production in women. Regular physical activity has been shown to lower endogenous estrogen production. You might be wondering, "Isn't estrogen important for women's health?" Yes, it absolutely is. But many women today face estrogen dominance.

This is due to environmental toxins, hormones in food, and some medications. Excess estrogen damages your body. It also increases your risk of cancer, particularly breast cancer. Exercise can help women lower their estrogen levels. It's like turning down the volume on a speaker that has been blaring too loudly.

The hormonal benefits of exercise extend beyond just one or two systems. Physical activity helps regulate a range of crucial hormones, including insulin, cortisol, growth hormone, and testosterone. It's akin to recalibrating your body's internal chemistry, ensuring all physiological systems are operating at their optimal levels. This hormonal recalibration can have wide-ranging effects—boosting energy levels, stabilizing mood, aiding in weight management, and enhancing cognitive function.

In my practice, I've seen the transformative power of exercise on hormonal health time and time again. Lisa was one of my patients who came to me struggling with symptoms of perimenopause—mood swings, hot flashes, and stubborn weight gain. We tried a comprehensive exercise program, rather than the commonly prescribed hormone therapy.

Within months, Lisa reported significant improvements in all her symptoms. Her mood stabilized, her hot flashes decreased, and she found it easier to maintain a healthy weight. This is the power of natural hormone regulation through movement.

Here's another crucial aspect of your health that doesn't get nearly enough attention: your lymphatic system. Think of your lymphatic system as your body's waste management and immune defense department. It's an intricate network of vessels and nodes that transport lymph, a fluid containing white blood cells, throughout your body.

Your circulatory system has the heart to pump blood, but your lymphatic system relies on movement to keep things flowing. Without movement, this critical system essentially grinds to a halt. It's like expecting your city's waste management to function without any garbage trucks on the road.

How does movement help? Each muscle contraction squeezes your lymphatic vessels, pushing the lymph fluid forward. It's like manually pumping a bicycle tire. The mechanics behind this process are simple yet essential. As your muscles contract and relax, they create pressure changes within the lymphatic vessels. These pressure differences open and close tiny valves in the vessels to ensure the lymph fluid flows one way and doesn't backtrack.

But it's not just about big movements. Even the simple act of deep breathing plays an important role in lymphatic circulation. A deep breath changes the pressure in your chest. It gently massages your thoracic duct, your largest lymphatic vessel. Think of it as providing a mini workout for your lymphatic system with every breath.

The benefits of better lymphatic function from exercise are remarkable. First, it helps maintain fluid balance in your body. This prevents the buildup of excess fluid (edema) in your tissues, reducing swelling and discomfort; similar to keeping all the pipes in your house clear and flowing freely.

Secondly, a well-functioning lymphatic system boosts your immune response. Your lymph nodes filter out pathogens and debris, allowing your white blood cells to fight infections better. It's a top-notch security system for your body, always on alert and ready to defend against invaders.

Lastly, regular movement lowers your risk of chronic inflammation. Chronic inflammation causes many health issues, such as arthritis and cancer. By keeping your lymphatic system flowing, you can put out inflammatory fires before they spread and cause lasting damage.

On the flip side, a sluggish lymphatic system can lead to many problems. When lymph fluid doesn't flow properly, toxins and metabolic waste can build up in your tissues. This can leave you feeling chronically fatigued and prone to headaches, with a weakened immune system. It's similar to living in a house where the garbage hasn't been taken out for weeks—everything starts to smell and functions poorly.

So, the next time you're considering skipping a workout or choosing the elevator over the stairs, think about your lymphatic system. Every movement, no matter how small, is an opportunity to support this crucial aspect of your health. A brisk walk, a yoga session, or deep breathing can help. These motions boost your lymphatic system, keeping you healthy and vibrant.

Rewire Your Mind with Exercise: The Fast Path to a Sharper, Happier You

You might think of exercise as something you do for your body, but it's time to recognize it as a powerful tool for your mental health as well. When you move your body, you're giving your brain a serious upgrade.

Let's start with the basics. Exercise increases blood flow to your brain by delivering oxygen and nutrients to your hardworking neurons. It's like giving your brain a spa day, complete with all the nourishment it needs to function at its best.

Exercise also stimulates a protein called brain-derived neurotrophic factor, or BDNF. Think of BDNF as fertilizer for your brain cells. It helps them grow, strengthens their connections, and even promotes the formation of new neurons. Neuroplasticity is key for learning, memory, and brain function. Every time you exercise, you're essentially giving your brain the tools it needs to rewire and improve itself.

Exercise is also a powerful shield against inflammation and oxidative stress. These harmful processes lead to the premature degeneration of your nerves. But regular exercise helps to preserve your brain and your mind for the long haul.

The benefits of exercise on your brain's health span your entire lifetime. For kids and teens, exercise boosts academic grades and brainpower. It's even strongly recommended for children with ADHD (attention deficit hyperactivity disorders) as a natural way to improve focus and attention. For adults, regular exercise helps maintain focus and mental sharpness. For older adults, staying active is a fountain of youth for the brain as well as the body. It helps prevent cognitive decline and preserves independence by reducing the risk of falls.

But perhaps the most exciting aspect is exercise's potential to prevent or delay the onset of neurological diseases. Take Alzheimer's, for example. This devastating condition is characterized by the buildup of harmful protein clumps in the brain. Exercise has been shown to reduce the formation of these clumps, providing a powerful defense against Alzheimer's. For those already diagnosed, regular exercise can help slow the disease's progression and improve cognitive function.

The same holds true for Parkinson's disease, which affects movement and coordination due to the loss of certain brain cells. Activities that boost balance, strength, and flexibility can help people with Parkinson's. They can improve motor function, reduce other symptoms, and may slow the progression of the disease. These activities can also make the brain more adaptable and resilient overall.

Every time you exercise, you're also triggering a cascade of feel-good chemicals in your brain. First up are endorphins, often called the body's natural painkillers. These powerful chemicals flood your system during exercise. They boost your mood and reduce your pain. Endorphins are your own cheerleading squad in your brain. They create a natural high that can leave you feeling euphoric and invincible.

But endorphins aren't the only mood boosters at play. Exercise also gives a boost to endocannabinoids and dopamine, both of which are part of your brain's reward system. Dopamine regulates your mood, motivation, and sense of pleasure. Physical activity prompts your brain to produce these feel-good chemicals, which can boost your enjoyment and satisfaction, making the activity more rewarding.

The mood-enhancing effects of exercise don't stop when your workout ends. Regular exercise can greatly improve your sleep by increasing the time you spend in deep sleep, the most restorative phase of the sleep cycle. This is like hitting the reset button for your brain, allowing it to recharge and repair itself more effectively. The result?

Enhanced brain function, more stable moods, and less stress—a balanced and resilient mental state.

If you're feeling stressed or anxious, exercise can also provide a constructive outlet for those feelings. It's a healthy way to burn off stress and excess energy. It helps with muscle tension and a racing heart. Plus, every time you complete a workout or reach a new fitness goal, you're giving your self-esteem and confidence a major boost.

Don't overlook the social benefits of exercise either. Group activities and sports can boost your well-being. They create a sense of community and belonging. Interacting with others during exercise combats loneliness and isolation. It also provides valuable emotional support.

In your mid-forties and fifties, it's more important than ever to shift from competitive exercise to fun, stress-reducing activities. This approach taps into the greatest longevity gains. Group physical activities can be a perfect and fun way to make this shift.

It's important to note that while exercise is a powerful tool for mental health, it's not a one-size-fits-all solution. The key is to find activities that you enjoy and that fit into your lifestyle. Whether it's dancing, hiking, swimming, or playing a sport, the best exercise for your mood is the one you'll stick with consistently.

Regular exercise boosts your physical health and nurtures your mind and emotions. You're stimulating your brain to keep it sharp and resilient, and finding a natural way to manage stress, boost your mood, and improve your quality of life. So, the next time you're feeling down or stressed, consider lacing up your sneakers and hitting the pavement. Your brain—and your mood—will thank you for it.

Get Stronger with Every Step: The Surprising Benefits of Daily Walking

For the perfect exercise, try walking. It's accessible, effective, and suits most people. It's the simplest form of physical activity, yet its benefits are profound and far-reaching. Whether you're eight or eighty, fit or just starting out, walking can be your gateway to better health.

Let's talk about what walking does for your brain. With each step, you're enhancing your brain's neuroplasticity, helping your brain to form and reorganize connections between neurons. This is especially true in response to new experiences and learning. The result is improved cognitive function, a brighter mood, and even reduced symptoms of anxiety and depression. It gives your brain a workout while you're on the move.

Walking is actually a full-body health booster. It helps regulate your blood pressure and keep it in a healthy range. The gentle, steady movement boosts your circulation and breathing. It lets oxygen flow better throughout your body. This, in turn, strengthens your heart and lungs, setting the stage for better health.

Here's something else that might surprise you: walking can be just as effective as running when it comes to cardiovascular health. I often recommend walking over running to my patients. This is especially true for those new to fitness or with joint issues. Walking is a low-impact exercise, so it puts less stress on your joints, but still provides great cardio benefits.

One of the best things about walking is that it can be easily incorporated into your daily routine. You can walk to work, take a stroll during your lunch break, or enjoy an evening walk with your family. And here's a tip: you don't have to do all your walking at once. Breaking it up into smaller sections throughout the day can be just as effective, if not more so. It's all about the total time spent walking, not one long, extended session.

I always recommend walking over other exercises, especially for beginners. It's better to walk for thirty minutes every day than to squeeze in a high-intensity workout once a week. Consistency is key when it comes to reaping the full benefits of walking.

Supercharge Your Health with the Power of Sunshine and Movement

If you're looking to supercharge your health, it's time to step outside. Combining sun exposure with physical activity is a powerful one-two punch for your well-being! It's not just about getting your daily dose of vitamin D or burning calories. This dynamic duo works together to boost your mental and physical health in surprising ways.

When you exercise outdoors, you're tapping into a natural mood booster that's hard to beat. Exercise releases endorphins. Sunlight boosts your mood. Together, they create a feel-good cocktail that can leave you energized and positive for hours—giving your brain a natural high, without any downsides.

The benefits go beyond just feeling good. Research shows that exercise and sun exposure can help prevent and treat Alzheimer's disease. Both exercise and vitamin D (produced by sunlight) are helpful, but the best results come from using them together. Activity boosts the nutrient's power to protect your brain.

Incorporating outdoor exercise into your routine doesn't have to be hard. Start by scheduling a morning walk or jog around solar noon when the sun is at its highest point in the sky. This ensures you're getting a healthy amount of sun exposure while also fitting in your daily movement. Aim for about twenty to sixty minutes of moderate outdoor activity several times a week. The exact amount will depend on your skin type and the climate. The key is to balance the amount of sunlight, without risking sunburn, to maintain healthy vitamin D levels.

If you're short on time, try breaking up your outdoor activity into smaller chunks throughout the day. Take a quick walk during your lunch break, have a standing meeting outside, or end your workday with a bike ride. Even simple activities count, like gardening or playing with your kids in the backyard. The goal is to make outdoor time a regular part of your routine.

Find Your Ideal Balance for Health—Exercise Smarter, Not Harder
What are exercise "sweet spots?" The answer might challenge some of the beliefs you have about exercise. The key takeaway is that more isn't always better when it comes to physical activity.

Let's start with moderate exercise, like brisk walking or leisurely cycling. Here's the good news: there's no upper limit to how much moderate exercise you can do. You could walk all day, every day, and you'd keep reaping health benefits. It's like a bank account where you can keep making deposits without ever hitting a maximum balance.

That's why I urge people to move more each day. They can take the stairs, park farther away, or have walking meetings.

But when it comes to high-intensity exercise, things get a bit trickier. Intense workouts have their place, but research shows that their benefits plateau after seventy-five minutes per week. That's right, just over an hour of high-intensity exercise per week is enough to see significant health improvements. Beyond that, you're not getting much additional benefit, and you might even lose some of the longevity benefits.

Despite all the well-known benefits of building muscle, the data clearly show that the benefits of strength training max out at forty to sixty minutes per week. That's not a typo. About an hour a week of strength training is all you need. Beyond that, you start to lose some of the benefits. This flies in the face of conventional bodybuilding wisdom, but the science is clear.

I've seen this play out in my own life. I had previously spent seven to ten hours in a fitness studio or my personal gym each week, doing intense strength training sessions. I even progressed to deadlifting over four hundred pounds at the age of sixty-eight. A 2022 paper I reviewed showed I was overexercising. I was getting little long-term benefit from all my effort. I now only do about three hours of resistance training a week.

A systematic review in the *British Journal of Sports Medicine* looked at sixteen studies. It found that muscle-strengthening activities were linked to a 10–17 percent lower risk of heart disease, cancer, diabetes, and death. Yet they found the maximum risk reduction was obtained at a dose of thirty to sixty minutes per week. After one hour, the benefits began to fade. At over 140 minutes per week, it raised the risk of death from any cause.

So don't push yourself to do high-intensity exercise for more than seventy-five minutes a week. Also, limit strength training to an hour or less, a few times a week. Doing more can work against you. If you're an overachiever by nature, focus that energy on moderate exercise instead. Remember, walking is a great moderate exercise. You can do it as much as you want, and you'll keep benefiting from it no matter how much you do.

The objective is balance. Yes, exercise is crucial for health and longevity, but more isn't always better. By finding your "sweet spot"—not too little, not too much, but just right—you can optimize your fitness routine. It will have maximum benefit and minimum risk. It's about working smarter, not necessarily harder, when it comes to your health and fitness.

Why Sitting Is the New Smoking: How to Break Free from Your Chair
You might think you're off the hook if you hit the gym regularly. Yet, as mentioned earlier, prolonged sitting will cancel out many of the benefits of your workout. That's right, even if you're a fitness enthusiast, spending hours glued to your chair is undermining your health. It's time to stand up (literally) for your well-being.

When you stand, you activate many muscles and cells in your body. You flip a switch that turns on your metabolism. Standing engages muscles throughout your body, from your legs to your core, keeping them active and burning calories. But it goes even deeper than that. Standing up activates processes that help regulate blood sugar, triglycerides, and cholesterol.

Sitting, on the other hand, is profoundly harmful to your health. Research links excessive sitting to over two dozen chronic diseases. We're talking about increased risks of heart disease, diabetes, certain cancers, and even depression. It's no exaggeration to say that sitting is the new smoking when it comes to health hazards.

But why is sitting so detrimental? One major factor is that it drastically reduces blood flow throughout your body. Just one hour of sitting can reduce blood flow to your main leg artery by up to 50 percent. This impaired circulation disrupts the systems that connect your blood to your muscles and tissues. That means elevated blood sugar, increased blood pressure, and higher cholesterol levels. It puts a kink in your body's fuel line.

So, what's the solution? Aim to sit for no more than about three hours a day total, and never for longer than fifty or sixty minutes at a stretch. I know this might sound impossible given the nature of many jobs today, but there are ways to make it work. One great option is a standing desk. If you're not used to standing all day, start small—just a few minutes per hour—and gradually increase the time. Remember, every little bit counts, and those small steps will add up.

Let me share a personal experience that really drove home the importance of reducing sitting time. For years, I struggled with persistent, nagging back pain that seemed impossible to shake. I tried everything under the sun to find relief. I visited chiropractor after chiropractor. I went through rounds of physical therapy. I experimented with photobiomodulation, which uses light to stimulate healing. I stretched until I felt like a rubber band. I hung upside down on inversion tables. And that's just scratching the surface. I probably tried a dozen other strategies that I can't even remember now.

But none of it worked. Not one of those approaches provided the relief I was desperately seeking. It was incredibly frustrating. Then, one day, it hit me like a bolt of lightning—the problem wasn't that I had a bad back, it was that I spent so much time sitting. I was clocking in anywhere from ten to sixteen hours a day in a chair, hunched over my desk. That's when I decided to make a radical change and switch to a standing desk.

The results were nothing short of miraculous. Within a brief time, the pain that had plagued me for years simply vanished. Now, I only sit when I'm traveling or when I'm feeling particularly tired. By addressing the root cause—excessive sitting—I finally found the solution that had eluded me for so long.

This experience was a powerful reminder that sometimes the simplest solutions can be the most effective. It's not always about finding the latest, most advanced treatment. Often, it's about looking at our daily habits and making simple changes that align with our body's natural needs. For me, that meant recognizing that my body is designed for movement, not prolonged sitting.

If you have back pain or other issues that resist treatment, consider how much time you spend seated each day. Sometimes, the key to better health is as simple as standing up and moving more. It certainly was for me, and it could be for you too.

Stand Tall: The Power of Proper Posture

Now that you're standing more, let's talk about how you stand. Your posture has a profound impact on your health and well-being, and it goes far beyond just looking confident. Proper posture optimizes your body's efficiency, reducing energy use and improving your nervous system's function.

Picture yourself standing tall, your head aligned with your spine, rather than tilted downward as many of us are prone to do. Your shoulders are relaxed and rolled back, allowing your chest to expand fully with each breath. Your hips remain level, avoiding any excessive tilt that could throw off your lower-back alignment. This is what proper posture looks like, and it's a game changer for your health.

By keeping this alignment, you promote good movement and lower your injury risk. But it goes deeper than that. Proper posture improves your energy expenditure. Think about it—when your body is aligned correctly, it doesn't have to work as hard to keep you upright and moving. This means you're using energy more efficiently, which can translate to feeling less fatigued throughout the day.

Proper posture also optimizes the signal transmission to your brain, enhancing your nervous system's efficiency. This improved communication translates into better coordination, balance, and physical performance. Suddenly, each step you take becomes a building block for better cellular health.

How can you achieve this ideal posture? Try sitting and standing tall, as if you're looking over a fence. This simple cue can help you maintain proper alignment and reduce the need for your body to compensate for poor alignment.

When your body mechanics are efficient, your muscles work in harmony, your joints move smoothly, and your body experiences less strain overall. This efficiency translates into reduced tightness, less pain, and a greater sense of ease and comfort in your daily life.

Here are a few additional practical tips to improve your posture:

- Imagine a string pulling you up from the crown of your head. This helps align your spine and neck.

- Keep your shoulders back and down, away from your ears. This opens your chest and improves breathing.

- Engage your core muscles. This supports your lower back and improves overall stability.

- When sitting, keep your feet flat on the floor and avoid crossing your legs.

- Take frequent breaks to stand, stretch, and reset your posture.

Remember, good posture is not about rigidity. It's about finding a natural, balanced alignment that allows your body to function optimally. It might feel awkward at first if you're not used to it, but with practice it will become second nature.

By combining increased standing time with proper posture, you're setting yourself up for optimal health. You're aligning your body for efficient movement, reducing strain and the potential for injury. You're also activating key cellular processes. This improves your metabolism and well-being.

So, stand up, stand tall, and give your body the alignment it craves. And remember, every slight change you implement adds up. You may not be able to change your routine overnight. But small, consistent gains in your standing time and posture can improve your health in the long run. Your body is designed for movement and proper alignment—it's time to honor that design and reap the rewards of better health and vitality.

Master Your Health Journey with the Right Tools at Your Fingertips

In our digital age, technology can be a powerful ally in your health journey. From simple step counters to advanced wearables, these tools can help you track your activity, sleep, and sun exposure. But as with any tool, it's important to use them wisely.

Let's start with the basics. Step counters and heart-rate monitors can be great motivators to get you moving more throughout the day. They provide real-time feedback on your activity levels, helping you set and achieve daily goals. Many find that seeing their step count can encourage them to take the stairs instead of the elevator or to park farther away.

Mobile phone apps offer a cost-effective alternative to dedicated fitness devices. These apps can use your phone's sensors to track your activity, sleep, and health. Some even have features to optimize your sun exposure. They alert you to the best times for vitamin D synthesis while minimizing the risk of overexposure.

However, it's crucial to be aware of the downsides of using your mobile device as a health tracker. Keeping your phone on you increases your exposure to EMFs, discussed in chapter 4. EMFs are mitochondrial toxins that can impact your cellular health. To reduce this risk, I recommend using airplane mode on your phone when tracking sleep or activity, especially at night. Airplane mode significantly reduces EMF emissions by turning off the device's cellular, Wi-Fi, and Bluetooth radios. This simple step can dramatically decrease your exposure to harmful electromagnetic radiation while still allowing you to use your phone's tracking features. By using airplane mode, you're essentially creating a safer environment for your cells to repair and regenerate, particularly during sleep when your body is most vulnerable to external stressors.

If you're looking for a dedicated fitness tracker, I often recommend the Oura Ring. Not only does it respect your personal data privacy, but it's impressive when it comes to sleep tracking. The ring tracks your sleep stage and its duration, using your body temperature, blood-oxygen levels, heart rate, and heart-rate variability. It tracks all stages of sleep, including light sleep, deep sleep, and REM sleep, giving you a comprehensive picture of your sleep quality.

One of the key benefits of using these tracking devices is the goal data they provide. It's easy to overestimate how much we're moving or how well we're sleeping. Having concrete numbers can help you identify areas for improvement and track your progress over time. Many of my patients are surprised to see how sedentary they are during the day, even if they consider themselves active. This awareness can be a powerful motivator for change.

It's important not to become fixated on the numbers. These devices are tools to help you understand and improve your health, not judgments of your worth. I always encourage my patients to use the data as a guide but also to listen to their bodies and trust their intuition.

I remember working with one of my employees, Richard, who became obsessed with hitting ten thousand steps every day. He would pace around his house late at night if he hadn't reached his goal, disrupting his sleep, and causing stress. We aimed to shift his focus. Instead of hitting an arbitrary number, he should move more naturally throughout the day. By making minor changes, like having walking meetings and doing yard work, he increased his activity without the added stress.

Used mindfully, these tracking devices can reveal your health patterns. They can help you identify trends, set realistic goals, and track your progress over time. These tools can help you along your path to good health. They can improve your sleep, increase your movement, and optimize your sun exposure by providing both data and motivation.

I also recommend downloading the Mercola Health Coach app if you haven't already. It integrates data from most of these apps. The app provides you with personalized analysis and recommendations to help you stay on track and achieve your health goals.

Remember, the goal isn't perfection, but progress. Every small step toward better health counts, whether it's tracked by a device or not. The most important thing is to find ways to move more, sleep better, and get safe sun exposure—whatever your lifestyle. Technology can be a helpful tool in this process, but it's your commitment to your health that will make the real difference.

 Scan this QR code to get FREE access to the Mercola Health Coach app. This tool allows you to log your meals, track your macronutrient ratios, and monitor your progress over time.

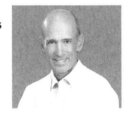

Nourish Your Body with Love: Why Embracing Healthy Carbs Can Transform Your Health

Your body is a marvel of biological engineering, with trillions of cells working tirelessly to keep you alive and thriving. The heart of this cellular symphony is the mitochondria. They are microscopic powerhouses that generate ATP, the energy currency of life. These structures are more than cellular components. They are the essence of your vitality and health.

Your cells hold an astonishing number of mitochondria, and they are hard at work. Each mitochondrion has about 2,500 ATP synthase enzymes, spinning at a mind-boggling five revolutions per second. There are an estimated 500 mitochondria in each cell, and about 40 trillion cells in the human body. That's a staggering 20 quadrillion mitochondria powering your existence at any given moment.

The scale of this energy production is awe-inspiring. These mitochondria collectively produce an unfathomable 200 million quadrillion ATP molecules every second. To put this in perspective, over the course of a single day, you produce the equal of your own body weight in ATP.

But the mitochondria's prowess doesn't stop at quantity. These tiny powerhouses are also incredibly efficient. In his book *Power, Sex, Suicide: Mitochondria and the Meaning of Life*, Nick Lane, PhD, a professor of evolutionary biochemistry at University College London, describes mitochondria as being a staggering ten thousand times more energy-dense than the sun itself. This efficiency lets your mitochondria meet the huge energy demands for constant cell and tissue repair.

Your body's energy production is huge because its requirement is so huge, so even a slight drop in ATP production can harm your health. It's not just that you're feeling tired, but that your body's ability to repair, regenerate, and defend against disease is at risk.

Your mitochondria's efficiency is literally the key to sustaining your life. Their rapid conversion of nutrients into ATP powers every vital function in your body, fueling muscle contractions, nerve impulses, and the synthesis of essential compounds. So, it's crucial to keep your mitochondria healthy to prevent and treat disease.

Bioenergetic Health Will Increase Your Energy and Help You Find Your Balance

In cancer research, few names stand out as prominently as Thomas N. Seyfried, PhD, a distinguished professor of biology, genetics, and biochemistry at Boston College. His work, based on the research of Nobel Prize–winning physiologist Otto Warburg, MD, PhD, is groundbreaking, challenging accepted views on cancer and its treatment.

Seyfried's seminal book *Cancer as a Metabolic Disease: On the Origin, Management, and Prevention of Cancer* offers a fresh perspective on this topic. At its core, he advocates a metabolic treatment for cancer, mainly focused on a low-carb diet, which he believed would starve cancer cells of their main energy source and slow their growth.

Seyfried's approach, while groundbreaking, has sparked significant debate in the scientific community, especially in comparison with the work of the late Ray Peat, PhD, a biologist and pioneer in bioenergetic medicine and human metabolism. Peat's bioenergetic principles, the basis of my Unified Theory of Cellular Health, offer a new way to view cellular energy and its role in health and disease prevention.

Peat's approach stresses the need for cellular energy, and challenges key components of the low-carb paradigm. According to Peat, a well-fueled cell can resist cancer because it can efficiently repair and regenerate. This view holds that carbohydrates are not the enemy but provide the vital energy your cells need for important tasks.

If you're feeling confused or even upset by this information, I completely understand. For years, many experts—myself included—advocated for minimizing carb intake as essential to health. Peat's views initially seemed so controversial to me that I consciously avoided engaging with them. My later realizations about the harm of vegetable oils and seed oils opened my eyes to the truth of his warnings.

As we explore cellular metabolism and ATP's role in health, we're on the brink of a new era in understanding disease and wellness. By supporting your mitochondria, you boost your energy. You also strengthen your body's defenses against many chronic diseases, including cancer. To be truly healthy and full of life, you must embrace a balanced approach. I've been in the health industry for decades, and I've seen countless diet trends come and go. But few have been as pervasive and enduring as the low-carb diet. I'll admit, I was once a staunch advocate of this approach.

My book *Fat for Fuel*, a number one bestseller, endorsed a low-carb ketogenic diet and fasting. I practiced what I preached, consuming fewer than 100 grams of carbohydrates daily, often dipping below 50 grams. I was convinced that carbohydrates were the enemy, something to be avoided at all costs. But we often underestimate the complexity of the human body. Our understanding of nutrition, mine included, is always being updated.

My journey toward a more nuanced understanding of carbohydrates and cellular energy began with a deep dive into Peat's work. His research on bioenergetics challenged many of my assumptions about low-carb diets. At first I was skeptical. After all, I had built a significant part of my career on promoting low-carb eating. But as I studied more of the science, I realized that there was much more to the story.

The idea that we don't need carbs is a dangerous oversimplification. The belief that your body can create all the carbs you need, though partially true, ignores the cost of making glucose from non-carb sources. This process, called gluconeogenesis, puts unnecessary stress on your body and can lead to a host of health problems. Sure, it will work for a while, but it's not sustainable or good for your body in the long run.

Many people fail to realize that a long-term, very low-carb diet will lower your ability to create cellular energy. This is why restricting carbs harms your health and longevity. Your cells need glucose—lots of it—to function optimally. When you deprive your cells of this essential fuel, you set the stage for metabolic dysfunction and disease.

This information might be hard to swallow, especially if you've been a devoted follower of the low-carb approach. Trust me, I've been there. It's not easy to change course after investing time, energy, and belief in a particular dietary philosophy. However, we must stay open to new ideas and adjust our practices when the evidence calls for it.

I hope my personal experience will help you overcome your fear of carbs. I want you to know that eating more carbs doesn't have to cause insulin resistance. When I initially slowly increased my carbohydrate intake from less than 100 grams to more than 500 grams, I noticed a slight increase in my weight—about five pounds.

But here's the surprising part: my body fat percentage decreased from 10 percent to 6 percent. You might wonder, "How is that possible?" The answer lies in improved metabolic efficiency. By providing my cells with more available glucose, my body became more efficient at using available nutrients for energy production.

It's time to question the prevailing low-carb dogma and explore a more balanced approach to nutrition. This doesn't mean swinging to the other extreme and consuming copious amounts of refined carbohydrates. Focus on whole, unprocessed sources of carbohydrates. Fruits, vegetables, and properly prepared grains are all part of a healthy diet that supports optimal cellular function.

Your body is a complex system that can heal and regenerate if given the right tools. A balanced mix of nutrients, including enough carbs, will support your body's natural ability to generate energy at the cellular level. This is crucial not just for day-to-day functioning but for long-term health and disease prevention.

As we explore cellular metabolism, we must rethink nutrition. We can't just label entire macronutrient groups as "good" or "bad." The story of cellular energy production is intricate and fascinating. It involves a delicate balance of several factors.

I hope that by sharing my journey and the insights I've gained, I can inspire you to think critically about your own approach to health and nutrition. The stakes are high, and the consequences of continuing to follow an overly restrictive dietary path can be severe. Using a balanced approach allows us to avoid the negative consequences of overly restrictive diets and instead work toward achieving true metabolic harmony.

Unveiling the Complex Truth behind Ketones and Sugar

As I dug deeper into the research on low-carb versus high-carb diets, I encountered another surprising finding that challenged the low-carb paradigm. Ketones, made in considerable amounts during ketogenic diets, can fuel cancer cells. This revelation calls into question the efficacy of ketogenic diets as a cancer treatment strategy. Cancer cells are very adaptable. We must match their sophistication in our treatments.

The Warburg effect, named after the Nobel Prize–winning physiologist Otto Warburg, is another crucial piece of the puzzle. Warburg observed that cancer cells tend to favor glycolysis for energy production, even when oxygen is plentiful. This observation has been widely misinterpreted as "sugar feeds cancer." But a more nuanced understanding reveals a different story.

The Warburg effect doesn't mean that cancer cells must burn sugar for fuel or that sugar inherently "feeds" cancer. Instead, it's more accurate to view cancer cells as damaged cells that can no longer normally metabolize glucose in their mitochondria. A range of factors have impaired their function. As a result, they are forced to rely on a less efficient form of energy production—burning glucose through glycolysis in the cytoplasm.

This inefficient energy production is a hallmark of cancer cells, but it's not the cause of cancer. Rather, it's a symptom of the underlying cellular damage. Focusing only on glucose misses the bigger picture: we must address the root causes of mitochondrial dysfunction and support cellular health.

A Breakthrough with Low-Carb Dogma and a Call for Balanced Metabolism

My growing knowledge of these complex cellular processes changed my views. I now recommend a different approach. This change faced resistance, especially from low-carb advocates I'd worked with and interviewed. Many struggled to consider an alternative viewpoint. The pushback I received highlighted a concerning trend in the fields of health and nutrition. Many influencers and experts become so invested in a diet that they resist new ideas that challenge their beliefs. I've seen this in the low-carb community. They treat the mantra "There is no minimum requirement for dietary carbohydrates" as gospel.

My studies have convinced me that a long-term low-carb diet is a recipe for metabolic disaster. It will reduce your ability to create cellular energy. In the long term, this approach will harm your health and shorten your life.

However, it's crucial to remember that everyone's nutritional needs are unique. I now recommend a higher carb intake for most people, but the best amount and types of carbs for you may vary. They depend on your health, activity level, and genes. As we study cellular metabolism, its complexities grow clear. Optimizing cellular energy production involves balancing several factors, including macronutrient intake, hormone levels, and toxic exposures.

You Need to Know Why the Bioenergetic Approach Offers New Hope for Cancer

Seyfried's research changed our view of cancer by challenging the belief that cancer is mainly a genetic disease. Seyfried proposes that cancer is a metabolic disorder driven by impaired mitochondrial function. This shift in perspective has transformed how we treat and prevent cancer.

Seyfried's theory says cancer cells have a unique metabolism. They rely on fermentation for energy, even in oxygen-rich environments. Seyfried argues that this metabolic shift drives cancer's growth and isn't just a result of it.

Based on this theory, Seyfried advocates for a treatment that targets cancer's metabolic weaknesses, especially by cutting carbs. The logic is simple: cancer cells need glucose to grow fast, so limiting glucose could starve them and slow tumor growth. This strategy underpins ketogenic diets for cancer treatment. They aim to shift the body's metabolism from using glucose to burning fat.

Seyfried's method shows promise in labs and clinics. But cancer is complex. No single approach will be effective for everyone.

Your Mitochondria Are the Overlooked Powerhouses for Preventing Cancer

The implications of Seyfried's seminal work extend far beyond cancer. His research shows that mitochondrial function is the key to cellular health and reveals the causes of many chronic diseases. Mitochondria are not just the cell's powerhouses—they are fundamental to cellular signaling, apoptosis (programmed cell death), and regulating the cell cycle. And compromised mitochondrial function can have far-reaching effects throughout the body.

Low mitochondrial energy production is now a factor in many diseases, including Alzheimer's, Parkinson's, heart disease, diabetes, and autoimmune disorders. Our understanding of how low-energy production causes disease is changing how we think about preventing and treating it, shifting our focus to strategies that support and enhance mitochondrial function.

In my clinical experience, I've seen massive health gains in people when they start focusing on mitochondrial health with targeted nutrition, lifestyle changes, and specific supplements. For example, Ellie, a thirty-five-year-old marketing executive suffering from fatigue and brain fog, saw significant improvements after adopting a mitochondrial health protocol. Key elements included daily niacinamide supplements, regular walks outdoors, and upping her carb intake.

> Within three months, Ellie reported increased energy levels, clearer thinking, and an overall boost in her quality of life.

When you look at cancer through the lens of cellular energy production, a new narrative emerges: cancer is a major disruption in cellular energy metabolism, not just rogue cell growth from genetic mutations. It emphasizes the need for strong mitochondrial health to prevent and treat cancer.

In healthy cells, mitochondria are energy sensors. They regulate metabolism and control cell division. When mitochondrial function is impaired, it creates a cascade of events that promote cancer development. Damaged mitochondria produce more reactive oxygen species (ROS) that cause oxidative stress and DNA damage. Damaged mitochondria may also fail to trigger apoptosis in cells that should die. This allows cancerous cells to survive and grow.

Seeing cancer as an energy problem, not just unchecked cell growth, opens new ways to intervene. It suggests that restoring normal mitochondrial function could be a powerful way to prevent and treat cancer. This could include diet, supplements, and lifestyle changes to boost mitochondrial health.

Although chemotherapy is a standard cancer treatment, it has limits and risks. Chemotherapy drugs target rapidly dividing cells, including many healthy ones. This is also the reason for many of its side effects, such as hair loss, nausea, and immune suppression.

But the damage caused by chemotherapy goes beyond what's visible. One of the most concerning aspects is its impact on the gut microbiome. Chemotherapy drugs hurt colonocytes, the rapidly dividing cells that line your intestines. Damage to these cells can cause "leaky gut," when the intestinal barrier is compromised such that toxins and undigested food can then enter the bloodstream. This can trigger widespread inflammation and many other health problems.

Moreover, chemotherapy fails to address the root cause of cancer. If we view cancer as a metabolic disease from faulty mitochondria, then chemo drugs will harm patients in the long run because they damage mitochondria. They may shrink tumors in the short term, but might cause new cancers by further harming cellular energy production.

This is not to say that chemotherapy never has a place in cancer treatment. In some cases, it can be lifesaving. But we must be more cautious in its use. We should weigh the benefits against the real, lasting damage it can cause.

Understanding That Healing and Not Destroying Cancer Cells Is the Answer

Cancer cells are not alien invaders. They are our own damaged and dysfunctional cells. This perspective changes how we approach treatment. Instead of viewing cancer as something we must attack and destroy at all costs, we can see it as a condition to correct and heal.

At the core of this cellular damage is the destruction of mitochondrial energy production. When cells' mitochondria can no longer produce energy, they rely on less efficient methods, like fermentation. This metabolic shift is a hallmark of cancer cells. It explains their rapid growth and ability to thrive in low-oxygen environments.

The inability of these damaged cells to repair and regenerate properly is another factor in cancer development. Normal cells have mechanisms to detect and repair damage or to trigger cell death if the damage is too severe. In cancer cells, these mechanisms often fail, allowing damaged cells to divide and accumulate more mutations.

Understanding cancer cells as damaged normal cells provides new avenues for treatment. Instead of just killing cancer cells, we can try to restore normal cell function by supporting the body's natural healing processes. This includes ways to improve mitochondria function, reduce oxidative stress, and support DNA repair.

In my practice, I've had success with a blend of methods that combines targeted nutrition, stress reduction, and select supplements to support cellular repair and regeneration. While these strategies are not a magic bullet, they are powerful tools within a holistic approach to cancer prevention and treatment.

As we continue to unravel the complexities of cancer metabolism, it's clear that our approach to this disease needs to evolve. By focusing on restoring normal cellular function, we may find better, less toxic treatments. The key is to address the root causes of cell dysfunction instead of just attacking cancer cells. Mitochondrial health is central to this because healthy mitochondria maintain cell integrity and prevent disease.

I've witnessed the devastating effects of chemotherapy far too many times in my friends, relatives, and employees. It's heartbreaking to see so many rush to oncologists, driven by fear or loved ones' pressure. They accept what I identify as "suicide chemotherapy." It's a choice, often made in panic, that frequently leads to a tragic outcome.

In my extensive experience, most of these individuals don't survive. What's even more distressing is that they often succumb not to the cancer itself but to the severe side effects of chemotherapy. A harsh truth, often ignored by the medical field, is this: chemotherapy is toxic; it destroys cancer cells, yes, but also healthy ones.

From what I've observed over decades in practice, choosing chemotherapy in most cancer cases is one of the worst choices a patient can make. It's not merely ineffective in many instances but it can also obliterate any hope of recovery. Chemotherapy often damages your immune system and gut microbiome to the point where they hinder your body's natural healing process.

The medical establishment pushes chemotherapy as their main treatment. It ignores or downplays alternatives that could be less damaging and more effective in the long run. Why? Follow the money trail and you'll find your answer. The cancer-treatment industry is a multi-billion-dollar behemoth with little incentive to explore treatments that can't be patented and sold at high prices.

Chemotherapy, the go-to treatment for most cancers, is fundamentally flawed. It's like using a sledgehammer to kill a fly on your kitchen table—sure, you might get the fly, but at what cost? The collateral damage is immense. Your immune system, the very thing you need to fight cancer naturally, takes a massive hit. It's a short-sighted approach that leaves patients at risk for recurrence or secondary cancers.

My recommendation? Explore every avenue before committing to a course of conventional cancer treatment. Don't let fear or pressure rush you into a treatment that could do more harm than good. Seek second and third opinions. Look for practitioners who are open to integrative and alternative methods. Your life may, quite literally, depend on it.

Remember, your body has an incredible capacity for healing when given the right support. Don't underestimate the power of natural, holistic approaches to cancer treatment. Alternative therapies garner less attention yet may provide a more effective route.

Beyond the Low-Carb Hype: Why Cutting Carbs Is Not Your Answer for Better Health

For decades, people have praised low-carb diets as the best way to improve blood sugar and insulin sensitivity. It's a compelling narrative: cut the carbs, lower your blood sugar, and voilà—insulin resistance solved! But if low-carb diets were a cure for metabolic health, we'd expect many people to benefit from them. After all, low-carb diets have been popular for decades, yet a staggering 99 percent of the US population is insulin resistant!

This paradox raises some crucial questions. If low-carb diets are so good at fighting insulin resistance, why haven't they improved our health stats? Is there a gap in our understanding of carbs, insulin, and metabolic health? The truth is that the link between low-carb diets and insulin resistance is more complex than many popular diet books claim.

Compelling research suggests that long-term low-carb diets make insulin resistance worse. This is due to a protective mechanism where your body preserves glucose for the brain by reducing its uptake in other tissues. This isn't necessarily harmful on a ketogenic diet, but it complicates our understanding of the long-term effects of carb restriction on metabolic health.

Cutting carbs can improve blood sugar for some in the short–term, but it's clearly not a one-size-fits-all solution to our metabolic health crisis. Our population's high insulin resistance points to deeper issues that go beyond just eating too many carbs.

Chronic stress, poor sleep, toxins, and nutritionally deficient, contaminated food harm our metabolism. These are often overlooked in the simplistic "carbs are bad" narrative. To tackle the insulin resistance epidemic, we must be holistic. We must consider not just our diet but also our lifestyle, movement, and environment.

Many health and fitness experts, including a growing number of medical doctors, recommend cutting carbs to lose weight. But the mechanism behind this approach is often misunderstood. The weight loss experienced on a low-carb or ketogenic diet is mostly water loss and muscle loss. As a result, people who stop these diets often regain lost weight, and their total body fat percentage does not change much.

More disturbingly, recent research shows that these diets can raise your risk of atrial fibrillation (A-fib). A-fib is a common heart arrhythmia that causes a rapid and irregular heartbeat and raises the risk of stroke and heart failure. This risk should worry those considering a long-term low-carb diet.

A-fib risk rises with age due to structural changes in the heart, such as thickening and stiffening of the heart muscle and the degeneration of the heart's electrical system. Aging also often brings other conditions such as hypertension, diabetes, obesity, and heart disease, which further raise the likelihood of developing A-fib. Atrial fibrillation affects millions worldwide. In the US, 2.7 to 6.1 million have it. So we must not ignore this potential side effect of low-carb diets.

At first glance, it seems logical to link metabolic disorders, like diabetes and obesity, to carbohydrate intake as these disorders are marked by high blood sugar levels. This has led many to mistakenly conclude that carbs cause high blood sugar. But this view ignores the true role of carbs, treating them as the enemy when they are essential energy sources for your mitochondria.

Carbs are like firefighters at a fire. They are there to extinguish the flames, not to ignite them. Similarly, carbs support your energy and balance your metabolism. When you see elevated blood sugar levels in conditions such as diabetes, it's easy to conclude that carbs are the problem. But this is akin to blaming firefighters for the existence of fires.

Understanding these nuances is key to making good adjustments to your health. The low-carb approach seems logical, but it oversimplifies the complex factors that affect metabolic health. Focusing only on carbs may overlook other key aspects of nutrition and lifestyle that are equally as important to our well-being.

Understanding the Real Culprits Behind Poor Metabolic Health

When discussing carbs and health, we must distinguish between whole and processed foods. Many health experts rightly blame processed foods for disease. But they often misplace the blame on the sugars in these foods. The real culprits are more harmful components, such as processed vegetable or seed oils.

Let's be clear: I'm not advocating for unlimited consumption of processed sugars. Processed sugars in high amounts can cause nutritional deficiencies. They provide calories but lack the essential micronutrients your body needs for metabolism. Over time, this can significantly impair your microbiome and biological health.

But it's crucial to differentiate between processed sugars and omega-6 fats, especially linoleic acid (LA). I believe the latter is far more damaging to your health. The real culprits in many processed foods are industrial seed oils, which are linked to inflammation and metabolic dysfunction.

If you eat mostly unprocessed, nutrient-rich foods, small amounts of sugar won't harm your metabolic health. However, this is contingent on maintaining a healthy microbiome. This caveat underscores the importance of focusing on a diet that supports gut health rather than vilifying specific nutrients.

Your brain is one of the most energy-demanding organs in your body. As stated in earlier chapters, although your brain only accounts for about 2 percent of your body weight, it consumes an astonishing 20 percent of your total caloric intake. This fact alone should give you pause when considering severe carbohydrate restriction.

Glucose, derived from carbohydrates, is your brain's primary and preferred energy source, so low glucose can harm your brain. It can even cause a life-threatening hypoglycemic coma. Your brain needs a constant supply of glucose to support vital functions, such as breathing, motor function, and heartbeat regulation.

This doesn't mean you need to constantly eat carbs, of course. Your body has clever ways to keep blood sugar levels steady, even when you fast or eat few carbs. But these mechanisms are designed for short-term adaptation, not as a long-term energy strategy.

During fasting or very low-carb diets, your body adapts. It produces ketones and lactate as alternative fuels for your brain. Let's break this down:

- Ketones are produced by your liver from fats when glucose is in short supply. These molecules can cross the blood-brain barrier and serve as an alternative energy source for your brain. Ketones can supply up to 70 percent of your brain's energy during long fasts or strict low-carb diets.

- Lactate, often seen only as a waste product of anaerobic metabolism, is an alternative fuel source for your brain. It's produced by your muscles and specific cells in your brain called astrocytes. Like ketones, lactate can serve as brain fuel when glucose is scarce.

While ketones and lactate can help when your glucose is low, they cannot fully replace carbs. Glucose remains necessary for full cognitive function and optimal metabolic activity. Some parts of the brain—for example, those involved in complex thinking—need glucose for peak performance.

This is why, even in states of ketosis or fasting, your body maintains a baseline level of blood glucose. It's a testament to the critical importance of glucose for brain function. Ketogenic diets and intermittent fasting can be beneficial in some cases, but they are not optimal long-term strategies for most people.

Your brain alone requires a minimum of 125 grams of carbohydrates daily. When you factor in the needs of your entire body, that number jumps to at least 250 grams per day. This isn't just my opinion; it's a biological fact that's often overlooked in our carb-phobic culture.

Let's consider your liver's role in this equation. In a healthy individual, the liver can store about 125 grams of carbohydrates as glycogen. But here's where things get concerning: the widespread use of processed seed oils has caused an epidemic of nonalcoholic fatty liver disease (NAFLD). It now affects 25 to 40 percent of the population. If you have NAFLD, your liver's ability to store glycogen can be diminished by as much as 50 percent.

Do the math and you'll see that for many people, their daily minimum carbohydrate requirement is likely north of 250 grams, just to meet basic needs. And that's before we even factor in exercise or other high-energy activities. This revelation flies in the face of many popular low-carb diets that restrict carb intake to less than 50 grams per day.

Let me share a personal anecdote to illustrate this point. After years of research and self-experimentation, I now eat 400 to 500 grams of carbs daily. Yes, you read that right. This is a far cry from my previous low-carb advice. I've seen big gains in my energy, brain function, and overall health since then.

But here's a crucial caveat: don't load up on carbs without first addressing your gut health. Most of us have altered and damaged microbiomes due to years of poor diet and lifestyle choices. Simply adding carbohydrates back into your diet without first healing your gut can make any disease symptoms you have far worse. Why? Because the carbs are feeding pathogenic, endotoxin-producing bacteria rather than good bacteria. Increasing carb intake is a complex issue that requires a personalized approach, which is why I have dedicated an entire chapter to this topic (see chapter 10, "Your Gut's Rainbow: A Simple Introduction to Carb-Fueled Gut Repair").

So, what happens when you don't eat enough carbs? On my low-carb fasting days, I saw a puzzling thing. After the second day of a water fast, my blood sugar levels spiked. This counterintuitive response is the body's clever adaptation to ensure survival. Without carbs in your diet, your body makes glucose from protein in your muscles and tissues.

This process, called gluconeogenesis, is triggered by stress hormones: glucagon, cortisol, and adrenaline. While it's a testament to your body's resilience, it's far from ideal as a long-term strategy. Gluconeogenesis is very inefficient. It takes a lot of energy to convert proteins into glucose. Also, gluconeogenesis causes muscle loss and a lower metabolic rate. This slower, more complex process is the opposite of what most people want from their diets. It does not provide energy as quickly or efficiently as consuming carbohydrates directly, which results in reduced performance and increased fatigue.

Gluconeogenesis is vital for survival in times of scarcity. But it should not be a routine strategy for health or weight loss. The energy-intensive nature of this process leads to a net loss of your body's energy stores. It's like running a business where the costs to produce revenue exceed the gross amount—a surefire path to bankruptcy.

Hopefully you can now begin to appreciate that it's better for your health to get glucose directly from carbs. This keeps your metabolism balanced and efficient. So, don't fall for the low-carb hype. Your body needs carbs, and denying it this fuel can have serious long-term consequences.

The Simple Power of Time-Restricted Eating Will Help You Feel Lighter and Energized

In recent years, scientists have explored the benefits of shorter fasting periods. They call it intermittent fasting or time-restricted eating (TRE). These approaches aim to harness some of the benefits of fasting while minimizing the risk of reductive stress.

The idea behind TRE is to limit your daily eating window to a specific timeframe, giving your body a consistent daily fasting period. This can boost your circadian rhythms and may improve metabolic health.

While the research on TRE is still in its early stages, some studies have shown promising results. It appears that TRE increases some beneficial gut bacteria and helps with weight and health. Below I list some simple points to consider when trying this approach.

- Limit meal frequency. Aim for three main meals a day instead of constant snacking.

- Restrict your eating window. Confine your eating to a twelve-hour period but not less than eight hours daily.

- Schedule your meals wisely. Begin eating shortly after you wake up in the morning. Finish your last meal at least three hours before bedtime to support better sleep.

One of the benefits of TRE is that it activates a powerful repair process called autophagy, which is your body's cellular cleanup system. Autophagy is a natural process that cleans out and recycles damaged cells, proteins, and organelles. By regenerating cells, autophagy helps prevent disease and promote longevity.

Of course, TRE isn't the only method for autophagy. Exercise is another way to clean up cells. Exercise lowers insulin levels, which is important because high insulin can stop autophagy. Another key player in the autophagy game is your thyroid gland. This tiny, butterfly-shaped gland in your neck makes hormones that greatly affect your metabolism and cellular function.

The two main thyroid hormones, T3 and T4, act like a turbo boost for your cells, revving up activities such as metabolism, energy production, and overall cellular function. But that's not all—thyroid hormones also stimulate the creation of new mitochondria. More mitochondria mean more energy production, which in turn supports more robust autophagy. It's a virtuous cycle that keeps your cells healthy and functioning at their best.

Feeling Stuck? Heal Your Microbiome First for a Stronger, Healthier You

As mentioned, before you jump on the high-carb bandwagon, you need to heal your microbiome. Increasing your carbs without fixing your gut is like trying to build a house on a shaky foundation. In chapter 10, I give detailed guidance on how to assess and improve your gut health. But first, let's review why this is so important.

Your gut is home to trillions of microorganisms that play a vital role in your overall health. These tiny microbes influence everything from your immune system to your mood and metabolism. When it comes to carbohydrate metabolism, the makeup of your microbiome is particularly important. Certain beneficial bacteria thrive on fibers in complex carbs. They produce short-chain fatty acids (SCFAs) that support gut health and reduce inflammation.

Optimizing your gut health involves promoting beneficial bacteria and limiting harmful, oxygen-tolerant bacteria. As beneficial, oxygen-intolerant bacteria begin to thrive, your carb metabolism will increase, allowing you to safely eat more complex carbs without skewing your microbiome in the wrong direction. When you get this balance right, you unlock the true potential of starch as a metabolic fuel. Your body can then efficiently convert carbs into energy without the negative side effects that many fear.

But this is not a one-size-fits-all approach. What works for me may not work for you, and vice versa. The key to success on a higher carb diet comes down to your gut health. If your gut health is poor, some carbs will cause nothing but problems. This is why it's crucial to take an individualized approach to your health journey. You need to listen to your body and pay attention to how it responds to different foods and eating patterns.

This means being mindful of how you feel after meals. Track your energy levels throughout the day. Track key biomarkers, like fasting blood glucose and fasting insulin. Your glucose level is easily measured and tracked at home using a glucometer, a small device that tests a drop of blood typically taken from your fingertip. Monitoring your fasting blood glucose levels can provide insights into how well your body manages blood sugar, which is a key indicator of metabolic health. A fasting insulin test is frequently included in routine bloodwork, or you can specifically request it from your health-care provider during routine checkups.

These indicators can tell you how well your body processes carbs and whether your current approach is improving your metabolic health. Don't be afraid to adjust based on what you observe. Your body is unique, and your diet should reflect that.

Approach your health journey with an open mind and a willingness to learn. Too often I see people get stuck in rigid thinking patterns, clinging to outdated information or fad diets that don't serve them. The field of nutrition is constantly evolving, and new research is emerging all the time. Stay curious, ask questions, and be willing to challenge your own assumptions.

Expect obstacles and setbacks along the way. The path to optimal health isn't always smooth or linear. There will be times when you feel like you're not making progress or when old habits creep back in. This is normal and part of the process. Just stay committed to your goals and don't let temporary setbacks derail you.

One of the best ways to stay on track is to surround yourself with a supportive community. This could be friends and family who share your health goals, a local wellness group, or an online community of like-minded people. Sharing your journey with others can provide motivation, accountability, and insights.

Your health is your most precious asset—without it, nothing else matters. Taking a proactive approach to your well-being now can save you from a world of pain and medical expenses down the road. It means making smart choices about your diet and lifestyle based on science, not fad diets or quick fixes.

Remember, every choice you make—from what you eat for breakfast to how much sleep you get—is an investment in your future health. It's about playing the long game, making decisions that will serve you not just today or tomorrow but for years to come. This might mean making some tough choices or breaking old habits, but I promise you, it's worth it.

As we wrap up this section, I want to leave you with some final words of encouragement. Trust in the process. The journey to optimal health is just that—a journey. It takes time, patience, and persistence. Don't expect overnight miracles. But do expect gradual, lasting gains in your health and well-being.

Be patient with yourself. Rome wasn't built in a day, and neither is optimal health. Celebrate the small victories along the way—every healthy meal, every workout, and every good night's sleep are steps in the right direction. These small steps add up over time, leading to considerable progress.

Remember, you have the power to transform yourself. By healing your microbiome, listening to your body, and staying open to new ideas, you can achieve vibrant health.

Lastly, I hope my journey and insights will inspire you. Question the dogmas. Explore a more holistic approach to nutrition and wellness. The stakes are high, and the consequences of continuing down an overly restrictive dietary path can be severe.

By providing your body with a balanced array of nutrients and listening to its needs, you can unlock your full potential for health and vitality. The journey to optimal health is ongoing, and I'm excited to continue learning and sharing new insights with you along the way.

CHAPTER 8

Love Your Cells: How Changing Your Oils Can Rapidly Boost Your Well-Being

Next time you're in the grocery store, take a closer look at the labels on those bottles of "vegetable oil." Soybeans, corn, and canola are grown in vast monoculture fields that stretch as far as the eye can see. The term *vegetable* conjures images of healthy, garden-fresh produce, making these industrial oils sound far more nutritious than they really are. It's a clever marketing ploy that's been fooling consumers for decades. I've visited these industrial farms, and let me tell you, they're a far cry from the idyllic scenes depicted on those bottles. Instead, these farms feature row after row of genetically modified crops, doused in pesticides and herbicides. It's a stark reminder of how disconnected we've become from our food sources.

The production process of these seed oils is equally concerning. Gone are the days of simple cold pressing. Today's seed oils are extracted using powerful machines and harsh chemicals, resulting in a substance that is more chemical than food.

But the food industry doesn't want you to know this. They use terms like "heart-healthy" and "cholesterol-free" to make these industrial oils seem like smart choices. It's a classic case of greenwashing—making something appear more natural and beneficial than it really is. As someone who has been fighting against these deceptive practices for years, I can tell you that it's all smoke and mirrors.

What's truly alarming is how ubiquitous seed oils have become. They're in almost every processed food you can think of—cookies, crackers, salad dressings, and even so-called health foods. It's a game of hide-and-seek where your health is at stake and the odds are stacked against you.

I've seen firsthand the transformative effect of eliminating seed oils from one's diet. Patients with chronic inflammation, weight issues, and cognitive decline have been able to slow, halt, or reverse these conditions. It's not always easy—these oils are everywhere—but the benefits are undeniable.

Break Free from Industry Manipulation and Use the Power of Natural Fats to Heal

To understand how we got here, we need to look back to the late nineteenth century, when food companies discovered they could produce cheap oils from crops like soybeans and corn, sparking a financial goldmine that would reshape global nutrition.

As the industry grew, so did its influence. It lobbied governments and health organizations, effectively shaping dietary guidelines to favor its products. The industry secured hefty farm subsidies for their crops, ensuring a steady supply of cheap seed oils, while traditional animal fats became more expensive. Perhaps most insidiously, it funded biased research claiming polyunsaturated fats were beneficial and saturated fats were harmful, further cementing seed oils' position in the market.

The postwar economic boom accelerated this shift. Urbanization led to increased demand for convenient, processed foods, which were packed with cheap seed oils.

Public health researcher Ancel Keys's "Seven Countries Study," which found a correlation between saturated fat intake and heart disease rates in seven diverse populations, became the cornerstone of the anti-saturated-fat movement and shaped dietary guidelines for decades. The American Heart Association endorsed these dietary changes, lending them medical credibility.

However, skepticism about Keys's hypothesis existed even before the study was fully published. For example, in 1957, statisticians Jacob Yerushalmy and Herman Hilleboe published a critique of Keys's earlier work, questioning his data selection and analysis methods. After the full publication of the "Seven Countries Study" results in 1978, more structured criticism began to emerge in the scientific community, including the claim that Keys excluded certain countries that didn't fit his hypothesis. When more countries were added, the link between saturated fat intake and heart disease disappeared. Still, the dogma that saturated fat causes heart disease lingers to this day.

The results of the seed oil industry's marketing and lobbying efforts were dramatic and far-reaching. Soybean oil consumption in the United States skyrocketed, increasing a thousandfold between 1909 and 1999. The average intake of linoleic acid (LA), the primary fatty acid in seed oils, more than doubled. This shift led to a significant change in the composition of the American diet, with LA comprising 7.21 percent of caloric intake as of 1999, up from just 2.79 percent in 1909. This unprecedented change in human nutrition represents a radical departure from traditional dietary patterns.

Today, the edible-oil industry is a behemoth controlling everything from seed development to product marketing. Consumers face a David-and-Goliath battle against misinformation and manipulation, but you have more power than you realize. By understanding the scope and influence of this industry, you can make informed choices about the fats you consume.

Break Free from Seed Oils: The Most Important Step to Recover Your Health

Let's get down to brass tacks. If you want to reclaim your health, you need to start by eliminating all vegetable and seed oils from your diet. I'm not talking about a gradual reduction; I mean a complete overhaul of your eating habits. Start in your own kitchen. Toss out those bottles of "vegetable" oil. When you eat out, ask what oils they use. If vegetable oil is the answer, either choose something else or ask them to cook your dish in butter. Be a food detective; always on the lookout for hidden seed oils.

Your goal should be to bring your LA intake down to 5 grams or less per day. This might sound drastic, but it's closer to what our ancestors consumed and what our bodies are adapted to handle. I know what you're thinking: "Dr. Mercola, that's impossible! These oils are everywhere!" You're right—they're in practically every processed food and almost everything you order at restaurants.

I've seen patients break down in tears when they realize just how prevalent these oils are. It can feel overwhelming, like you're swimming against an impossible current. But I'm here to tell you that it's not only possible to cut these oils from your diet, it's essential for your health.

So, what's the alternative? Let me introduce you to some old friends that have been unfairly demonized: tallow, butter, ghee, and coconut oil. These traditional fats that have nourished humans for millennia are packed with nutrients your body craves. Tallow is rich in vitamins A, D, and K2. Butter—especially from grass-fed cows—is one of the lowest sources of LA and is brimming with beneficial fatty acids.

I remember the first time I reintroduced butter into my diet after years of avoiding it due to misguided health advice. The flavor was a pleasant surprise, but even more impressive were the health benefits I experienced. My energy levels soared, my skin improved, and I felt more satisfied after meals. It was a powerful reminder that our bodies know what they need—we just have to listen.

But it's not just about switching out your cooking oils. You also need to be aware of other significant sources of LA in your diet. Whole seeds and nuts, while nutritious, can be loaded with LA. And don't get me started on conventionally raised chicken and pork. These animals are typically fed LA-rich corn and soy, resulting in meat that is exceedingly high in LA.

I've visited farms where chickens are raised on these LA-rich feeds, and the difference in meat quality is stark. The fat is softer, more prone to oxidation, and lacks the nutrient density of traditionally raised poultry. It's a vivid illustration of how the seed oil industry's influence extends far beyond the obvious sources.

Cooking Oils	% Linoleic Acid (LA) Average Value (Range in Parentheses)
Safflower	70%
Grape seed	70%
Sunflower	68%
Corn	54%
Cottonseed	52%
Soybean	51%
Rice bran	33%
Peanut	32%
Canola	19%
Olive oil	10% (3% to 27%)
Avocado	10%
Lard	10%
Palm oil	10%
Tallow (CAFO)	3%
Ghee/Butter (CAFO)	2%
Coconut oil	2%
Tallow (Grass Fed)	1%
Butter (Grass Fed)	1%

Comparative analysis of the linoleic acid (LA) content in various cooking oils and fats, arranged in descending order. Linoleic acid, an omega-6 polyunsaturated fat, is represented as a percentage of the total fat composition. The oils are color-coded, showing various levels of LA content: red, high LA content; orange and yellow, moderate LA content; green, low LA content.

When it comes to beef, there's an interesting twist. The difference in LA content between grass-fed and grain-fed beef is minimal—only about 0.5 percent. But don't let that fool you into thinking it doesn't matter. Grass-fed beef is better because it's usually lower in contaminants, such as glyphosate, antibiotics, and hormones.

Also, let's talk about salmon for a moment. The farmed variety, which makes up most salmon consumed today, is a nutritional disaster. It's high in harmful fats, low in beneficial omega-3s, and loaded with contaminants. I've seen lab reports that show PCB (polychlorinated biphenyl) levels in farmed salmon that are eight times higher than in wild salmon. It's a stark reminder that farmed and wild fish are not interchangeable in terms of nutrition and health impacts, so choose wisely.

We face a harsh reality: the edible-oil industry has reshaped our food system. It affects the crops we grow, the animals we raise, and the products on our store shelves. It's sobering, but understanding the scope of the problem is the first step toward reclaiming your health. In the face of this industrial onslaught, your choices matter more than ever. Every meal is an opportunity to push back against this nutritional disaster and nourish your body the way nature intended.

Once you start eliminating LA from your diet and embracing traditional fats, you'll experience a profound shift in your relationship with food. You'll rediscover the joy of cooking as your dishes explode with flavor and the satisfaction of a meal that truly nourishes your body. You'll start to see food not just as fuel but also as medicine.

I've seen this transformation in many of my friends. They come to me frustrated, confused, and often sick. But as they cut seed oils and embrace traditional fats, their health improves dramatically. Chronic inflammation subsides. Weight issues resolve. Many report better mood and thinking.

Are you ready to take control? To break free from the grip of Big Food and rediscover what real, nourishing food tastes like? It starts with a single step—eliminating those seed oils from your plate.

Seeds/Nuts	% Linoleic Acid (LA) Average Value (Range in Parentheses)
Poppy seed	62%
Hemp	57%
Wheat germ	55%
Walnut	53%
Pecan	50%
Pumpkin	45%
Brazil nuts	43%
Sesame	41%
Peanut	32%
Pine nuts	33%
Chia	16%
Almond	16%
Flaxseed	14%
Pistachio	13%
Hazelnuts	12%
Cashew	8%
Macadamia	2%

Comparative analysis of the linoleic acid (LA) content in various nuts and seeds, arranged in descending order. The nuts and seeds are color-coded, showing various levels of LA content: red, high LA content; orange and yellow, moderate LA content; green: low LA content.

Rethink Your Fats, as Overusing "Healthy" Oils Will Sabotage Your Health

I have a story that will astonish you. For years, we've been told that olive oil and avocado oil are the pinnacle of healthy fats. But what if I told you that these so-called superfoods might do more harm than good? It's time to pull back the curtain on a health myth that's been making us sicker.

First, let's talk about what's really in that bottle of olive oil you've been drizzling over your salads. Studies show over 90 percent of the bottles are adulterated with cheap seed oils. In 2017, a Taiwanese food mogul was sentenced to two years in prison for selling olive oil that turned out to be 98 percent palm oil. So, chances are you're not getting pure olive oil but a cocktail of industrial oils masquerading as a health food. Even if you're lucky enough to get your hands on the real deal, you're still not out of the woods.

Olive oil and avocado oil are packed with monounsaturated fats (MUFAs), particularly oleic acid. We've been told these are healthy fats, but the truth is more complicated. Like LA, when consumed in excessive amounts, MUFAs can wreak havoc on your mitochondria. They lead to a buildup of lipid intermediates, such as ceramides and diacylglycerols, which disrupt cellular membranes and block the transport of key molecules in and out of the mitochondria.

But it gets worse. These MUFAs can increase fat deposition in tissues that aren't meant for fat storage, like your liver and muscles. This impairs mitochondrial function and reduces the efficiency of energy production. In simple terms, you're reducing ATP production—the energy your body needs to function properly.

I know what you're thinking: "But Dr. Mercola, hasn't olive oil been linked to improved cholesterol levels and reduced heart disease risk?" You're right, and that's where things get tricky. Moderate use can be helpful for heart health, provided the olive oil is truly pure. But too much is harmful.

Your body has a sophisticated system for processing fats, including the ability to convert one type of fat into another. When you consume too much oleic acid from these supposedly healthy oils, you're not just adding this fat to your body but also encouraging your body to produce even more of it from fats you already have stored.

The bottom line? While olive oil and avocado oil aren't as harmful as industrial seed oils, they're far from the health panaceas we've been led to believe. Moderation is key, and it's crucial to approach all foods—even those with a health halo—with a critical eye. For years, we've been told that the Mediterranean diet, which is rich in olive oil, is the gold standard for health. But what if I told you that Greece, Spain, and southern Italy—Mediterranean countries that consume a lot of olive oil—have some of Europe's highest obesity rates? It's true, and it's a paradox that's had me scratching my head for years.

I'm not saying olive oil is the enemy, but we need to look at the whole picture. Olive oil has polyphenols, powerful antioxidants that mask the harmful effects of oleic acid. It's quite likely that these polyphenols, not the fat itself, are responsible for many of olive oil's touted health benefits.

This illustrates a key point: even healthy foods can be bad in large amounts, making moderation the key. I've seen too many patients who thought they were right to douse everything in olive oil and then battled weight gain and metabolic issues.

Let's talk about saturated fats. You've probably been told to avoid them like the plague. But hear me out. Saturated fats are rarely converted into inflammatory by-products in your body. Why? It's all about their chemical structure. They lack the double bonds that make fats such as LA vulnerable to oxidation, a critical step in the formation of inflammatory mediators.

Take coconut oil, for example. It's rich in medium-chain triglycerides (MCTs), a type of saturated fat that's a true nutritional powerhouse. Unlike other fats, MCTs bypass the usual storage process in fat cells and are transported directly to your liver and quickly converted into energy. This means that MCTs can help with weight management rather than contribute to fat gain.

In obese people, body fat is mainly polyunsaturated fats (PUFAs), not saturated fat. Why? Because saturated dietary fat is mostly burned and used for energy, rather than being stored. It's the excessive consumption of LA that leads to its accumulation in fat cells.

The animal agriculture industry has known about this for decades. In fact, they have been using this knowledge to fatten up livestock more efficiently. Studies from the early twentieth century proved that pigs fed saturated fats, mainly coconut oil, became lean and muscular, but pigs fed PUFAs gained mostly fat. This led to the widespread use of PUFAs in animal feed. The goal was to maximize "caloric efficiency"—to get the animals as heavy as possible using as little food as possible.

Recent animal research has also shown that maternal overconsumption of LA raises the risk of obesity in offspring. The researchers think the intergenerational effect may be due to changes in the offspring's gut microbiota. Excessive LA consumption seems to cause intestinal inflammation and gut barrier dysfunction, which allows obesogenic bacteria to thrive.

This is why I'm so passionate about reducing LA intake. It's not just about your health but also the health of future generations. Our metabolism is remarkably similar to that of pigs. So it's no surprise that as we eat more PUFAs, we struggle with obesity.

What's the takeaway here? It's time to rethink our relationship with fats. Don't be afraid of saturated fats from healthy sources like coconut oil or grass-fed animals. Be mindful of your olive oil consumption, and for heaven's sake, steer clear of those industrial seed oils. I've developed a tool called Food Buddy on the Mercola Health Coach app that can help you track your LA intake. It's incredibly precise, telling you how much omega-6 you're getting from your food down to the tenth of a gram, and about 90 percent of that omega-6 is LA.

Choosing Low-PUFA Foods Will Improve Your Health and the Planet

Let me paint you a picture of how PUFAs and MUFAs work together to damage your health. Think of PUFAs as the bullet: they're the primary culprit in causing inflammation and metabolic dysfunction. MUFAs are the trigger. While not as directly harmful, they set the stage for PUFAs to do their damage. It's a one-two punch that's been knocking out our health for decades.

However, we can change this. It starts with supporting farmers who use low-LA feed for their livestock. I've seen firsthand the difference this can make. Take the Michigan-based regenerative farmers Ashley Armstrong, PhD, and her sister, Sarah, for example. They've started a chicken farm network that's producing eggs with 80 percent less LA than commercial eggs. That's not just a small improvement—it's a game changer.

But the Armstrongs aren't stopping there. They're on a mission to train other farmers across the United States to produce not just low-PUFA eggs but also chicken and pork. This is the kind of grassroots movement that can transform our food system from the ground up.

To understand why this is so important, you need to know a bit about how different animals process fats. Ruminants such as cows, lambs, goats, and deer have a unique digestive system that converts dietary PUFAs into saturated fats. It's like they have their own built-in fat processing plant. But monogastric animals—chickens, pigs, and, yes, humans—do not have this ability. Whatever fats we eat get directly incorporated into our tissues.

This is why conventionally raised chicken and pork are often so high in PUFAs. To make matters worse, many conventional farmers are now using dried distilled grains (DDGs), which are waste products from the ethanol industry, in their animal feed. DDGs raise the PUFA content in livestock even further.

Industrial farmers are even trying to use technology to turn the naturally occurring saturated fats in ruminant animals into PUFAs. This is seriously misguided. They're deliberately sabotaging the healthiest source of saturated fat left in our food system.

Once you understand the pervasive presence of LA in your diet, you can start making informed choices. Every meal is an opportunity to nourish our bodies and shape the future of our food system. By supporting regenerative farmers who focus on low-PUFA animal products, you're helping to shift the entire food system toward more sustainable, health-promoting practices.

Every time you choose a low-PUFA option, you're telling producers, retailers, and policymakers that this is what consumers want. In a market-driven system, that's a powerful message. So, join the food revolution and make every bite count.

CHAPTER 9

Awaken Your Inner Vitality: How Collagen Can Gently Build and Transform You

While most people associate protein primarily with building muscle mass, these remarkable molecules, composed of amino acids, play a far more comprehensive role in our health. Dietary proteins are the primary building blocks of your body's structure and function. They form the foundation of not just muscles but also bones, cartilage, and skin.

Beyond structural support, proteins promote cognitive function and longevity. In the brain, they aid neurotransmitter production, aid in cell repair, and help maintain cognitive flexibility, all of which contribute to keeping your mind sharp as you age.

When it comes to longevity and disease resistance, muscle mass acts as a powerful shield against many health issues. High muscle mass helps you fight heart disease, cancer, and nonalcoholic fatty liver disease (NAFLD). Dietary protein, especially from animal sources, is indispensable to building and maintaining this muscular armor.

Protein also supports cellular repair throughout your body. It bolsters your immune system and helps maintain metabolic health, which are important factors in aging well.

The impact of prioritizing protein in one's diet can be transformative. As a specialist in nutritional medicine, I hold a fellowship from the American College of Nutrition. Throughout my career, I have lost count of how many times I have seen optimizing protein intake transform someone's digestive health. The transformation is particularly evident in patients struggling with bloating, irregular bowel movements, or poor nutrient absorption. These individuals often experience significant improvements when they incorporate the right type and amount of protein into their diets.

I've also witnessed people reverse their diabetes diagnosis and sharpen their memory and focus, all by ensuring adequate protein intake. I've found that the answer lies not just in increasing protein consumption but in tailoring protein intake precisely to each patient's needs.

Conversely, the impact of muscle loss can be devastating. Cachexia, a severe loss of muscle mass, affects up to 80 percent of cancer patients and contributes to a staggering 20 percent of cancer deaths. By focusing on protein intake and muscle preservation, we can help cancer patients maintain their physical and mental health, giving them that much more of a fighting chance as they battle disease.

Muscle Mass Supports Your Health at Every Stage of Life

Your muscles are a primary reservoir for amino acids. For this reason, having high muscle mass is imperative when you're sick, because your body's demand for these building blocks rises dramatically during recovery from illness or injury. I've seen patients recover much faster by maintaining good muscle mass through proper nutrition.

Muscles also play a vital role in regulating your metabolism and managing glucose disposal. This makes them essential in controlling conditions such as diabetes and heart disease.

As you get older, maintaining adequate protein intake becomes even more critical. It is your best weapon against sarcopenia, the natural loss of muscle mass that comes with aging. I've worked with many older adults who thought weakness and frailty were inevitable. But by eating more protein and doing resistance training, they've regained strength, improved their balance, and rediscovered their zest for life.

Eating enough protein also boosts your metabolism and maintains healthy bones. This means you're not only staying strong but also keeping up your energy levels and reducing your risk of fractures. It's a powerful combination that can dramatically improve your quality of life as you age.

At the most fundamental level, dietary protein is essential for the function and regeneration of every single cell in your body. This includes your immune cells, which rely on protein to mount an effective defense against pathogens and other threats. Patients with chronic infections and weak immune systems often do not recover. I knew many people who fit this description during the COVID-19 pandemic, and it's likely their protein deficiencies put them at a greater disadvantage.

Because the protein you eat affects your muscles, organs, immune system and cells in general, I always stress to my patients the importance of choosing high-quality sources. It's not just about quantity— the type and quality of protein you consume can make a world of difference in your health.

Calculating Your Protein Needs

Let's talk about how much protein you really need. The magic number is 0.8 grams of protein per pound of ideal body weight—meaning not your current weight but rather the weight you would ideally be based on your height, age, and gender. There are several ideal body weight calculators online that are easy to use. Just plug in your age, gender, and height and the calculator will give you a range based on commonly used formulas.

Next, calculate your daily protein requirement. For example, if you weigh 160 pounds but your ideal weight is 128 pounds (the equivalent of having 20 percent body fat), you'd multiply 128 by 0.8, giving you a daily protein target of 102.4 grams.

The figure you arrive at might seem like a lot, but when spread out over your meals, it's totally doable. In the example provided above, that's about 33 grams per meal if you're eating three times a day. Here are two examples of meals that would provide you with that amount of protein:

- Five ounces grilled wild-caught salmon (30–35 grams of protein) with 1 cup roasted Brussels sprouts (about 3 grams of protein).

- Four ounces grilled top sirloin steak (about 23 grams of protein), served with 1 cup cooked broccoli (4 grams of protein), 1/2 cup cooked spinach (2.5 grams of protein), and 1 cup cooked Brussels sprouts (3 grams of protein).

Feel Healthier with Protein: The Key to Boosting Your Energy and Immune Function

Think of protein as the raw material your body uses to build its defense forces. Protein is essential for creating immune cells. Without enough protein, your immune system is like an army without weapons or armor. Take lymphocytes, for instance. These little warriors, including T-cells and B-cells, are the special forces of your immune system. They need protein to make cytokines, which are chemical messengers that coordinate your immune response. B-cells use protein to make antibodies, your body's custom-made defense against specific invaders.

Macrophages, your immune system's cleanup crew, also rely on protein to create enzymes that help them find and destroy pathogens. Neutrophils, your first line of defense against infections, use protein to make powerful microbe-killing enzymes. And let's not forget about natural killer (NK) cells, your body's "assassin squad." NK cells rely on protein synthesis to produce the necessary enzymes, receptors, and signaling molecules that identify and destroy infected or abnormal cells.

Protein also keeps you energized and oxygenated. It is essential for creating hemoglobin, the star player in your red blood cells. Hemoglobin is like a microscopic delivery truck, picking up oxygen in your lungs and dropping it off wherever your body needs it.

Without enough protein, your body struggles to produce hemoglobin. This leads to a decrease in functional red blood cells, leaving you feeling tired and weak. I've seen patients complaining of constant fatigue, and low protein intake is often the culprit.

Those red blood cells, packed with hemoglobin, deliver oxygen to your mitochondria. This oxygen is crucial for the mitochondria to convert nutrients into ATP, the energy currency of your body. So, by ensuring you have enough protein, you're not just supporting your blood—you're fueling every single cell in your body.

Eating protein also slows down your body's absorption of sugar during digestion, which prevents rapid spikes in blood sugar that can leave you feeling jittery one moment and exhausted the next. If you struggle with energy crashes throughout the day, increasing your protein intake might make a world of difference.

Protein stimulates the gradual, controlled release of insulin from the pancreas. This steady insulin response helps maintain consistent blood sugar levels over time. It's like having a thermostat for your blood sugar, keeping everything in the optimal range.

Protein also triggers the release of glucagon, a hormone that works opposite to insulin. When your blood sugar starts to dip, glucagon tells your liver to release stored glucose, stabilizing your energy levels. This balance of insulin and glucagon, controlled by protein, provides a steady energy supply all day.

And let's not forget that protein is great at promoting satiety. That feeling of fullness and satisfaction after a meal helps prevent overeating and stabilizes blood sugar levels. It's a win-win situation for your energy and your waistline.

Let's look at how protein supports your digestive system. It's not just about what protein does for you after it's digested; it plays a crucial role in the digestive process itself. Protein helps regulate the pace at which food moves through your digestive tract, allowing time for nutrient absorption and preventing heartburn, indigestion, and other common digestive complaints.

In your stomach, the presence of protein activates enzymes such as pepsin, which breaks down the protein into smaller components. Pepsin also stimulates gastrin secretion, a hormone promoting stomach acid production. This acid is needed for proper digestion and the absorption of nutrients.

As the partially digested food moves into your small intestine, protein continues its work, stimulating the release of pancreatic enzymes which are vital for breaking down proteins, fats, and carbohydrates. This ensures that you're getting the most out of all the nutrients in your meal.

As the protein continues to be digested, it is broken down into amino acids, which are then absorbed into your bloodstream and transported throughout your body. Your cells reassemble them in countless ways to create new proteins that serve a wide variety of functions, from building muscle tissue to creating enzymes and hormones.

I often use the analogy of LEGO blocks to explain amino acids to people. Just as you can build countless structures with LEGO, your body uses amino acids to construct the proteins it needs for various functions. This simple concept makes it easier to grasp why dietary protein is so important for your overall health.

Feeling Weak? Essential Amino Acids Can Boost Your Strength and Mood

Essential amino acids are the VIPs of the amino acid world. Your body can't produce them on its own, so you must get them from your diet. There are nine essential amino acids: histidine, isoleucine, leucine, lysine, methionine, phenylalanine, threonine, tryptophan, and valine.

Each of these amino acids plays a unique role in your body, including tissue repair, immune function, hormone production, and energy metabolism. In my years of practice, I've seen deficiencies in these essential amino acids lead to a wide range of health issues.

Getting enough of these amino acids isn't just about avoiding deficiency; it's about optimizing your health. I've had patients enjoy remarkable improvements: their energy, muscle strength, and well-being all increased once they got enough essential amino acids.

Histidine, for instance, is involved in tissue growth and the production of both red and white blood cells. Patients with anemia often improve significantly once their histidine intake is addressed.

Isoleucine and leucine work together to support muscle metabolism and repair. They're particularly important for athletes and anyone looking to maintain or build muscle mass. And because leucine plays a role in blood sugar regulation, it is also beneficial for managing diabetes.

Lysine is a key player in protein production and growth. It also aids calcium absorption, making it important for bone health. I've had great success using lysine supplementation to help patients with osteoporosis.

Methionine is vital for tissue repair and detoxification, but you need to be careful with methionine. Excess methionine has been linked to decreased longevity. It's a perfect example of why balance is so necessary in nutrition.

Phenylalanine is a precursor to several important neurotransmitters. It's fascinating how this single amino acid can influence your mood, focus, and cognitive function. I've seen great improvements in patients suffering from depression and ADHD once they optimized their phenylalanine intake.

Threonine supports the digestive tract and is therefore vital for nutrient absorption and gut health. In my practice, I've found that fixing threonine deficiency can be a game changer for patients with digestive issues.

Valine is another muscle-supporting amino acid that plays a role in energy production. It's particularly important for endurance athletes and anyone dealing with fatigue.

Lastly, there's tryptophan. It's involved in protein synthesis and immune function, but like methionine, it requires careful balance. Tryptophan is a precursor to serotonin. While many people have heard of serotonin, few understand its complexities.

Serotonin isn't the "feel-good" neurotransmitter it's often made out to be. In fact, elevated serotonin levels can be problematic. I am cautious about recommending tryptophan supplements or selective serotonin uptake inhibitors (SSRIs) because they increase serotonin levels.

High serotonin levels can lower your metabolic rate and contribute to obesity and fibrosis. It's a classic example of how mainstream medicine often oversimplifies complex biological processes. I've seen patients struggle with weight gain and other health issues due to serotonin-boosting interventions.

The issues with elevated serotonin don't stop there. Elevated serotonin inhibits pyruvate dehydrogenase (PDH), an important enzyme for energy production in your mitochondria. When serotonin puts the brakes on PDH, it causes less efficient ATP production. This is why many people on SSRIs experience fatigue and weight gain. Lastly, let's discuss conditionally essential amino acids, which become essential in certain situations, especially during illness or stress. This group includes arginine, cysteine, glutamine, tyrosine, glycine, ornithine, proline, hydroxyproline, and serine. Arginine is important for immune function and wound healing. I have used arginine supplementation successfully with patients recovering from surgery.

Glutamine is particularly interesting. It's a primary fuel source for immune cells and intestinal cells. However, like many things in nutrition, balance is key. Excess glutamine can cause problems, particularly in people with an unhealthy gut microbiome, including the overgrowth of harmful bacteria, which may worsen dysbiosis and cause gastrointestinal issues such as bloating and diarrhea. Excess glutamine can also exacerbate intestinal permeability, contributing to leaky gut and triggering inflammation or autoimmune responses. Additionally, excess glutamine can cause imbalances in neurotransmitter levels, triggering neurological issues such as anxiety or migraines.

Glycine: The Unsung Hero of Amino Acids

Glycine, another standout conditionally essential amino acid, is involved in the production of glutathione, one of your body's most powerful antioxidants. This amino acid is a true multitasker in your body, and its benefits are nothing short of remarkable. In animal studies, glycine has been shown to extend lifespan—in some cases, it has even increased median lifespan by up to 28.4 percent. That's not just adding years to life but life to years.

Glycine is a powerful anti-inflammatory agent. I've recommended glycine supplements to patients with chronic inflammatory conditions from arthritis to heart disease. The results can be dramatic: reduced pain, improved mobility, and better health.

When it comes to wound healing and gut health, glycine is a milestone of innovation. It helps repair and maintain the gut lining, which is crucial for optimum health. I've seen many with leaky gut syndrome improve remarkably just by increasing their glycine intake.

Glycine also plays a vital role in supporting liver and kidney function. These organs are your body's main detox systems. For patients with liver or kidney issues, glycine intake is key to recovery.

One of the most interesting aspects of glycine is its ability to suppress seizures and even tumors. It does this in part by inhibiting angiogenesis, the formation of new blood vessels that feed tumors. While more research is needed, the potential here is exciting.

Many people struggle with getting sufficient high-quality sleep, and glycine can be a natural solution for that as well. Glycine helps improve sleep quality without the side effects associated with sleep medications. Glycine has also shown promise in alleviating neuroinflammation and protecting against cognitive deficits. This could have huge implications for preventing and managing neurodegenerative diseases. I'm closely following the research in this area as it could be a breakthrough for brain health.

Lastly, glycine helps reduce the effects of excess tryptophan and serotonin, including free radical damage, inflammation, and cell death from ATP depletion or calcium overload. It also assists in preventing mitochondrial damage. It's like an internal repair kit for your body.

How Amino Acid Restriction Can Help You Live Longer

Glycine also plays a role in the effects of amino acid restriction on longevity. Amino acid restriction involves limiting specific amino acids in your diet to achieve certain health effects. This is possible because foods contain varying amounts of different amino acids, allowing selective reduction of some while still getting others. While caloric restriction has long been linked to increased lifespan, recent studies suggest that selectively limiting specific amino acids may yield even more impressive results.

Methionine restriction in particular has shown remarkable outcomes. Studies in rodents have demonstrated increases in lifespan ranging from 29 to 43 percent when methionine is restricted—a significant extension of life by any measure. Interestingly, research has also revealed that a high intake of glycine can mimic the life-extending effects of methionine restriction, offering a more practical approach to achieving similar benefits. This is why I'm so passionate about promoting a balanced approach to protein intake. By eating collagen-rich proteins that are high in glycine and low in methionine, you mimic the benefits of methionine restriction, avoiding the need for extreme diets.

From Inflammation to Sleep: The Many Ways Glycine Can Improve Your Life

Collagen is far more than just a buzzword in the beauty industry. It's a fundamental building block of your body's structure and function. Collagen is your body's most abundant protein. You may not realize it but one-third of the protein in your body is collagen. It keeps your skin, bones, and connective tissues strong and elastic. But its importance goes even deeper, right down to the cellular level.

I've been fascinated by collagen's role in our health for years, and my research has led me to some surprising discoveries. One of the most intriguing is collagen's relationship with structured water, also known as "gel water," within your body. This structured water is essential for cellular hydration and function, and the integrity of your cells' environment largely depends on having enough collagen to maintain this state.

You might be wondering why we're suddenly facing a collagen crisis when our ancestors seemed to do just fine. The answer lies in how dramatically our diets have changed over time. In the past, human diets were high in collagen because people typically ate every part of the animal.

Let's take a culinary world tour to see how different cultures used to incorporate collagen-rich foods into their diets. In many Asian countries, bone broth was (and still is) a staple. This nutrient-rich liquid is made by simmering bones for a long time, which breaks down the collagen and releases it into the broth. If you've ever had a bowl of authentic pho, you've experienced the rich, gelatinous texture that comes from this process.

Hopping over to Europe, we find dishes like aspic—a savory jelly made from meat stock. It might not sound appetizing to modern palates, but this collagen-rich dish was once considered a delicacy. In North America, Indigenous peoples practiced nose-to-tail eating. They ate not just the muscle meat but also the organs and other collagen-rich parts of the animal.

African tribes have long consumed the whole animal. They eat everything, including the tendons and ligaments, which are high in collagen.

These examples all point to a common theme: our ancestors didn't let any part of an animal go to waste. In doing so, they inadvertently ensured a steady supply of collagen in their diets. Fast-forward to today and the picture looks quite different, at least for Western cultures. The typical Western diet has shifted away from collagen-rich foods in favor of muscle meats and processed foods, which are low in or void of collagen.

Amino Acid	% Gelatin Collagen	% Beef
Glycine	28%	1.6%
Proline	17%	1.0%
Hydroxyproline	14%	0.3%
Alanine	11%	1.3%
Methionine	0.8%	3.2%
Histidine	0.8%	2.1%
Tryptophan	0.4%	1.3%
Cysteine	Trace	0.2%

Amino acid composition of collagen compared to that of beef protein.

How Collagen Harnesses Sunlight to Boost Your Energy

Let's explore a fascinating aspect of collagen that many experts overlook: its role in photometabolism. Collagen acts like a natural solar panel in your body. It collects and converts near-infrared radiation from the sun into usable energy for your mitochondria. I'm conducting research to prove that near-infrared light creates structured water, or "gel" water, when it interacts with collagen. This isn't your ordinary H_2O—it's a special form that acts as a transducer, converting solar energy into electrical potential.

Think of it like this: the structured water created by collagen becomes a kind of biological battery. It collects electrons in the space outside your cells and then releases them. Your cell membranes' transporters then pick up these electrons and shuttle them into your mitochondria. This process feeds directly into the electron transport chain, which is how your cells produce energy.

This mechanism could explain why sunlight exposure is so foundational for health, beyond just vitamin D production. It's a direct way for your body to harness the sun's energy. So, by optimizing your collagen intake and sun exposure, you can drastically improve your energy and overall health.

Most People Don't Get Enough Collagen: Why It's So Vital for Your Health

The numbers paint a stark picture. Current estimates suggest that the average American's daily collagen intake from food is alarmingly low, at just 3 to 5 grams. Even for those who consume greater amounts of foods like sausage and frankfurters—foods that often contain a higher level of collagen-rich animal parts—collagen intake is still low: an average 12.7 grams for women and 22.6 grams for men.

You might be thinking, "Well, that doesn't sound too bad." But these averages are too low to support healthy collagen production and cell maintenance. Ideally 25 to 30 percent of your total protein intake should come from collagen or gelatin sources. That's about 40 to 50 grams a day for most people.

The deficiency of collagen in our diet is further compounded by other aspects of our modern lifestyle. One factor that often gets overlooked is our limited exposure to natural sunlight. Sunlight plays a crucial role in vitamin D production, which in turn supports collagen synthesis. Plus, the infrared light from the sun can stimulate collagen production in your skin.

So, what's the solution to this collagen conundrum? One of the easiest and most effective ways to boost your collagen intake is by regularly consuming bone broth. I remember the first time I made bone broth—the rich aroma filled my kitchen, and I was amazed at how simple it was to prepare. If you're short on time, there are also high-quality collagen supplements available. Just be sure to choose ones derived from grass-fed, pasture-raised animals for the best nutritional profile.

Remember, every cell in your body is surrounded by a collagen matrix. Getting enough of this crucial protein gives your body the building blocks it needs for repair, regeneration, and optimal function. It's a simple step that can have profound effects on your health and well-being.

When it comes to getting the most bang for your buck in terms of protein quality, not all meat cuts are created equal. You might be surprised to learn that some of the less popular cuts, like oxtail and shanks, are nutritional powerhouses. These cuts are rich in connective tissue, which translates to a higher collagen content and a more balanced amino acid profile.

The first time I cooked oxtail, I was skeptical about this tough-looking cut. But the slow-cooked result was delicious and satisfying. Oxtail is rich in glycine, proline, and hydroxyproline, which are crucial for collagen production in the body. Shanks, whether from beef or lamb, are similarly rich in these collagen-forming amino acids. These cuts give your body the raw materials it needs to help maintain and repair your connective tissues.

And the bonus for those of us on a budget? These cuts are often cheaper than prime cuts like steak or chicken breast. It's one of those rare instances where the more affordable option is nutritionally superior. By incorporating these cuts into your diet, you're saving money and investing in your health.

Cooking these tougher cuts requires a bit more time and patience, but the payoff is worth it. Slow-cooking methods, such as braising, make the meat tender. They also break down the collagen into more digestible forms, which means your body can more readily absorb and use these valuable amino acids.

Confused About Collagen and Gelatin? Learn the Key Differences for Better Health

What's the difference between collagen and gelatin? It's a topic that often confuses people, but understanding the difference can help you make better choices for your health. At their core, collagen and gelatin have the same basic amino acid composition. They're essentially two forms of the same thing, but with some key differences in how they behave and how your body processes them.

Collagen is the raw form, the structural protein found in animal connective tissues. Gelatin is what you get when you cook collagen. Think of it like this: collagen is the tough, fibrous stuff that holds meat together, while gelatin is what makes your bone broth gel when it cools.

The production of gelatin involves heating collagen, which breaks down its molecular bonds. This process, known as partial hydrolysis, results in shorter protein chains. When you dissolve gelatin in water, it forms a thick gel. This is why gelatin is so popular in cooking and food production. This gel consistency is what gives gelatin desserts their distinctive wobble and thickens sauces and gravies.

But the benefits of gelatin go far beyond culinary applications. Because of its partially broken-down structure, gelatin is incredibly easy for your body to digest and absorb. When you consume gelatin, your body quickly breaks it down into its component amino acids and puts them to use.

Gelatin's high absorption makes it ideal for people with digestive issues and for those wanting a quick collagen boost. I often recommend gelatin to patients recovering from surgery or injury because its building blocks are readily available for tissue repair.

Gelatin is also useful for those with ulcers or gut issues. It coats and soothes the digestive tract, helping to heal the gut lining. I've seen patients with chronic digestive issues find relief by adding gelatin-rich foods or supplements to their diet.

But don't dismiss collagen just yet. Collagen supplements often come in a hydrolyzed form. They've been partially broken down to improve absorption, making them nearly as easy for your body to use as gelatin.

Understanding how collagen is produced can help you appreciate why it's such a valuable supplement. The process starts with animal parts rich in collagen—typically bones, skin, and connective tissues. These aren't the parts we typically eat, which is part of why our modern diets are so deficient in collagen.

The collagen extraction process involves treating these animal parts with either an acid or an alkali solution, which helps isolate the collagen from other components. What's interesting is that this process doesn't involve heat, which can denature proteins, changing their structure and effectiveness.

The result of the collagen extraction process is a substance with a larger molecular structure than gelatin. Because of this structure, collagen doesn't dissolve in water. If you've ever tried to mix collagen powder into cold water, you've probably noticed it doesn't disappear like other powders might. This is because its molecular structure is too large to dissolve fully.

Collagen's larger structure is both a blessing and a curse. Although it can provide more sustained support to your body's tissues, it is slightly harder for your body to break down and absorb. That's why many collagen supplements are processed to break them down into smaller peptides, which improves their bioavailability.

When it comes to health benefits, collagen and gelatin are remarkably similar. This shouldn't be surprising given that they're essentially the same thing in different forms. Both provide the same amino acids, and your body uses them to build and maintain connective tissues, support joint health, and keep your skin youthful.

It's important to remember that when you ingest collagen or gelatin, your body breaks it down in your gut into shorter peptides. These peptides are then further broken down into individual amino acids. It's these amino acids that your body uses for various physiological processes.

Ultimately, once absorbed, collagen and gelatin have the same effects. Your body doesn't care if the glycine and proline came from collagen or gelatin. It just uses them wherever they're needed.

Both forms have been linked to a wide range of health benefits. They may improve skin elasticity, reducing the appearance of wrinkles. They may reduce pain and stiffness in osteoarthritis. They can support joint health, improve gut health, and promote better sleep.

The choice between collagen and gelatin often comes down to personal preference and how you plan to use it. Collagen is more versatile—it can be added to both hot and cold liquids without changing their texture. Gelatin will cause liquids to gel, which can be great for making healthy gummies or thickening soups but might not be ideal for your morning coffee. If you want a daily supplement that won't change your food or drinks, collagen might be more convenient.

However, I can't stress enough how important it is to choose your supplements wisely. The supplement industry is largely unregulated, and not all products are created equal. Look for companies that are transparent about their sourcing and manufacturing processes. Opt for collagen from grass-fed, pasture-raised animals whenever possible. And always check for third-party testing to ensure purity and potency.

Boost Your Collagen the Fun Way: Homemade Gummies, Marshmallows, and More

The idea of drinking bone broth or taking collagen supplements might not appeal to everyone. But don't worry, I've got some creative and delicious alternatives that'll make boosting your collagen intake a breeze. One of my favorite methods is making homemade gummies or marshmallows using gelatin powder. It's a fun activity that the whole family can enjoy, and it's a sneaky way to get more collagen into your diet.

The first time I made homemade gummies was with a friend's kids. Their eyes lit up as we mixed natural fruit juices with high-quality gelatin powder, poured it into fun molds, and waited eagerly for them to set. We had a blast. I felt good, too. I was giving them a tasty treat, but unlike store-bought snacks, these weren't loaded with added sugars and artificial ingredients.

Making your own marshmallows is another great option. They're surprisingly easy to whip up, and you can control the sweetness and flavors. I like to use honey or maple syrup instead of refined sugar and add natural flavors such as vanilla or cocoa. The result is a fluffy, delicious treat that's packed with collagen-boosting gelatin.

But a word of caution: don't be fooled by commercial "gelatin" products such as Jell-O. You might be shocked to learn that Jell-O-brand snacks contain no gelatin at all. Instead, they use a substance called carrageenan, which is derived from seaweed. While that might sound natural and healthy, it's anything but. Carrageenan has been linked to inflammation and can contribute to a wide variety of chronic diseases. It also causes digestive side effects in many people.

Even Jell-O powder, which does contain some gelatin, is far from ideal. It lists sugar as the first ingredient and is full of artificial colors and questionable preservatives. These are exactly the kinds of processed foods that are wreaking havoc on our health. I cringe when I think about how many children are consuming these products regularly.

A pure gelatin powder without any additives ensures you get the full benefits of the gelatin without any harmful extras. Trust me, once you start making your own gelatin-based snacks, you will never want to go back to the store-bought versions. They're both healthier and tastier.

So, boosting your collagen intake doesn't have to be a chore. From homemade gummies to slow-cooked meats, there are many tasty ways to get enough of this vital protein.

Collagen and Muscle Meat: A Balancing Act

Now let's talk about why balancing your intake of muscle meat and collagen is so crucial for metabolic health. This is where many people, including health professionals, go wrong. They focus solely on muscle meat as a protein source, not realizing the potential downsides of this imbalanced approach.

Muscle meats are rich in certain amino acids like cysteine, methionine, and tryptophan. While these are essential, consuming them in excess can lead to inflammation and suppress your thyroid function.

I've seen countless patients with unexplained inflammation and thyroid issues. Their protein intake was too high in muscle meats.

On the flip side, collagen amino acids are like nature's antiaging compound. The key is to mimic the protein composition found in whole animals, which our ancestors consumed. Aim for about one-third of your protein intake to come from collagen or collagen amino acids.

This balanced approach to protein intake supports your body's structural health. It boosts energy and improves brain health. It can lengthen lifespan and improve your quality of life. It's a simple change that has profound effects.

The Egg Dilemma: A Protein Powerhouse with a Catch

We've talked quite a bit about the benefits of protein found in collagen, but no discussion of protein is complete without talking about eggs. Eggs are truly a nutritional marvel. They're an excellent source of high-quality protein and contain a wealth of nutrients that are hard to find in other foods. One of the standout nutrients in eggs is choline, found abundantly in the yolk.

Choline is a nutrient that doesn't get nearly enough attention, in my opinion. It's crucial for optimal brain function, it supports nervous system health, and it plays a role in eye health. It's also vital for cell structure, mitochondrial function, and metabolism. In fact, a 2020 study found that choline reduces inflammation. It can help those with insulin resistance or metabolic syndrome.

If you're not getting choline from other sources, you need to eat three to four egg yolks per day to meet your body's needs. If you're very active, you might need even more to support your higher metabolic rate. Ninety percent of Americans do not meet their choline requirements and, currently, supplementation with choline is not recommended as existing supplements all have problems.

But here's where things get tricky. Though eggs are nutritional powerhouses, conventional eggs have a big drawback: they're high in linoleic acid (LA). This is due to the LA-rich feed given to conventionally raised chickens. Why is this a problem? Well, it's been clearly shown that eggs high in LA can increase oxidized LDL cholesterol and boost your risk of heart disease.

To put this in perspective, one large conventional egg has about 0.7 grams of LA. If you're eating three eggs a day (which, remember, is what you need for optimal choline intake), you're already at 2 to 3 grams of LA. Ideally you want to keep your total LA intake below 2 grams per day.

Finding eggs that are low in polyunsaturated fatty acids (PUFAs) will take some effort, but it's well worth it. You might need to look beyond your regular grocery store and seek out local farmers or specialty markets. Talk to the farmers about their chicken-feed practices. You're looking for farmers who know that low-PUFA feed is key. These birds are often fed a diet more closely resembling what they'd eat in nature—insects, seeds, and greens. When you find a good source of low-PUFA eggs, stock up! These eggs allow you to reap all the amazing benefits of egg consumption without the drawbacks of excess LA.

Remember, when it comes to nutrition, quality is just as important as quantity. It's not just about how many eggs you eat but what *kind* of eggs they are. By choosing wisely, you can turn your morning omelet or scrambled eggs into a powerful tool for optimizing your health.

The Quest for Quality Animal Protein

The quality of your protein matters. Animal proteins are called "complete" proteins because they have all the essential amino acids your body needs in the right proportions. This makes them incredibly valuable for everything from muscle repair to enzyme production.

But modern farming methods have changed the nutrition of many animal products. The way animals are raised and what they're fed significantly affects the quality of the protein and fats in their meat, eggs, and milk.

This is why I always tell my readers to be selective about their animal protein sources. Protein from nonruminant sources such as pork and chicken can be problematic. These animals are often fed diets high in corn and soy, which lead to meat that is high in inflammatory omega-6 fats. For these meats, use only certified low-PUFA options.

Your best bet? Focus on ruminant animals such as cows, lambs, goats, and deer. These animals are designed to eat grass, and when raised properly, their meat tends to have a much healthier fat profile. It's lower in inflammatory omega-6 fats and higher in beneficial omega-3s.

But don't stop at just choosing the right type of animal. Look for grass-fed and pasture-raised options whenever possible. These animals live more natural lives and eat their natural diets, which makes their meat more ethical and nutritious.

Another important tool that can help you choose high-quality meat is the Digestible Indispensable Amino Acid Score (DIAAS). This powerful tool assesses the true nutritional value of different protein sources.

The DIAAS is a relatively new method that is replacing older, less accurate ways of measuring protein quality. What makes it special? It considers not just the amino acid profile of a protein source but also how well your body can actually digest and use those amino acids.

Here's how it works: Scientists measure each essential amino acid in a food and compare it to a reference profile based on human needs. Then they assess how well each amino acid is digested, typically measured at the end of the small intestine. This gives us a clear picture of how much of each amino acid the body can absorb and use.

Why does this matter? Because not all proteins are created equal. You might eat a food that's high in protein, but if your body can't efficiently digest and use those amino acids, you're not getting the full benefit.

This is where animal proteins often shine. Eggs, dairy products, meat, and fish typically score high on the DIAAS scale because their amino acid profiles closely match human needs. Our bodies digest and use these proteins efficiently.

But don't just take my word for it. Start looking for DIAAS information on food labels and in nutritional databases. Some forward-thinking companies are starting to include this information on their product labels, often listed as a percentage or a numerical value next to protein content. They recognize its value to health-conscious consumers like you.

Top Picks for High-Quality Animal Protein

So, what should you be putting on your plate? Here's a list of my top recommended sources of animal protein:

1. Beef from grass-fed cows or bison is rich in protein, B vitamins, and minerals such as iron and zinc. Ground beef is the least expensive and healthiest form of beef as it is typically made with connective tissue loaded with collagen.

2. Dairy products from A2 milk, and cheese made with animal rennet, are rich in calcium. Unlike traditional milk, which has both A1 and A2 proteins, A2 milk is produced by cows with specific genetics to yield only the A2 type of beta-casein protein. A2 milk protein is easier to digest for many people.

3. Goat and lamb are often naturally grass-fed and rich in nutrients.

4. Venison is a lean protein source that is high in iron and B vitamins.

5. Bone broth is packed with collagen and minerals that are great for gut health.

6. Low-LA eggs have all the benefits of eggs without the inflammatory omega-6 overload.

7. Wild-caught, low-fat fish, such as cod and sole, are high in protein and omega-3s and low in contaminants.

8. Collagen and gelatin support skin, joint, and gut health.

9. Shellfish are rich in zinc, selenium, and other trace minerals.

Is Your Cheese Safe?
The Hidden Dangers of Genetically Modified Rennet

Let me share a personal story that highlights the importance of being vigilant about what's in your food. A few years after having my mercury fillings removed, I noticed my kidney function was deteriorating. My creatinine levels were consistently above the normal range, sometimes spiking alarmingly high.

At the time, I was consuming large amounts of cheese—I'm talking five-pound blocks of mozzarella in less than a week. I loved the stuff! But I noticed that these cheese binges coincided with spikes in my creatinine levels. Through careful self-monitoring, I realized that cheese was somehow harming my kidneys.

It wasn't until years later that I discovered the likely culprit: synthetic rennet made with genetically modified organisms (GMO). In the early 1990s, cheese makers began using fermentation-produced chymosin (FPC), a cheap substitute for traditional animal rennet. By the mid-1990s, it dominated 80–90 percent of the commercial cheese market in the US and Europe.

Here's the problem: making this GMO rennet involves genetic modifications and industrial fermentation. These can produce harmful by-products, such as mycotoxins and endotoxins, that often make their way into the final cheese product—and from there, into your body.

Over time, cheese made with this GMO rennet can cause toxins to build up in your body, particularly in your kidneys. It can lead to oxidative stress, inflammation, and cell damage. This impairs kidney function and reduces your body's ability to produce energy.

What's troubling is that, in 1990, the FDA granted "Generally Recognized as Safe" status to this GMO rennet, seemingly prioritizing industry profits over public health.

The "safety" of FPC was evaluated by a single 90-day trial in rats. That means a single short-term study on rats is being used to justify the widespread use of this genetically modified enzyme in our food supply. FPC raises many safety concerns as it contains biotoxins and allergens from the host microorganisms used in production. These residues can cause digestive and respiratory issues and disrupt gut health. Also, there are no long-term studies on genetically modified enzymes.

What can we do about that? Just like you need to search for low-PUFA eggs, be proactive about your cheese choices. Look for cheeses made with traditional animal rennet. These can be harder to find and might cost a bit more, but your health is worth it. Read labels carefully. Many companies mislead you by calling GMO rennet "plant based." It's actually derived from genetically altered E. coli bacteria and is a clever form of greenwashing.

The protein sources you choose, from eggs to meat to cheese, are vital. They will protect your health and boost your nutrition.

Remember, every bite is an opportunity to nourish your body, so choose wisely!

Want Healthy Seafood?
Learn How to Choose Fish That Boosts Your Nutrition

Seafood is a fantastic source of protein as long as you vary the types of seafood you eat and know where it comes from. This approach ensures a diverse nutrient profile and reduces your exposure to any single contaminant.

For example, in my opinion, it's best to avoid farm-raised fish entirely. Farm-raised fish are often given diets that bear no resemblance to what they would eat in the wild. This leads to a nutritional profile that's significantly inferior to their wild counterparts. Plus, they're more prone to contamination from the crowded conditions they're raised in. I've seen lab reports comparing wild-caught and farm-raised fish, and their nutritional content is starkly different.

Instead, I recommend focusing on shellfish and warm-water finfish such as cod and sole. These options are low in fat and especially low in PUFAs. They're also less likely to accumulate heavy metals. Remember, heavy metals tend to be stored in fat, so leaner fish are generally a safer bet.

The Hidden Dangers of Eating Too Much Meat: Phosphorus and Iron Excess

Here's an often overlooked aspect of eating animal proteins: balancing your intake of phosphorus and iron. These minerals are abundant in meats, especially organ meats. While essential for your health, too much of a good thing can become problematic.

Phosphorus helps form bones and produce energy, but too much upsets the balance of calcium in your body. This imbalance can cause many health issues, including bone loss, premature aging, a higher risk of obesity, and heart problems.

I've seen patients who ate a lot of animal protein, especially organ meats, develop these issues. Their blood tests showed high phosphorus and low calcium, resulting in muscle weakness, bone pain, and kidney problems. The key is to maintain a proper calcium-to-phosphorus ratio, which according to medical literature should be between 1:1 and 1.3:1.

Iron is vital for making red blood cells and oxygen transport, but too much iron is a silent killer. It promotes oxidative stress and has been linked to a range of chronic health conditions, including heart disease and cancer.

In my practice, I always check patients' ferritin levels, which is a marker of iron stores in the body. Ideally you want your ferritin level below 100 ng/mL, preferably around 20–40 ng/mL. A level above 100 ng/mL typically indicates inflammation, high iron, or both. Anything above 200 ng/mL is considered pathological.

When your body absorbs more iron than it needs, it doesn't have an easy way to get rid of the excess. Over time, this extra iron builds up in your organs, especially in the liver, heart, and pancreas. This accumulation happens slowly, often without any obvious symptoms, making it a silent threat.

One of the biggest dangers of excess iron is that it leads to oxidative stress. Imagine it as your body's version of rusting from the inside out. This process harms your cells and tissues, and may lead to serious conditions like heart disease, liver damage, and diabetes. Also, high iron levels help harmful bacteria and viruses to thrive. This raises your infection risk and makes it harder to fight.

Some people are more at risk of iron overload, including those with genetic conditions such as hemochromatosis, which causes the body to absorb too much iron from food. Postmenopausal women and men are also at higher risk because, without regular blood loss, iron levels can accumulate over time. Also, frequent blood transfusions may result in excess iron in the body.

What makes excess iron particularly dangerous is how it builds up over the years. Regular blood tests allow you to monitor your iron levels effectively. If needed, making dietary adjustments, such as reducing red meat intake and donating blood, will help keep your iron levels in check.

Screening for iron excess begins with a simple blood test to measure your serum ferritin levels—that is, the amount of iron stored in your body. This test is the most reliable way to identify if your iron levels are in the triple digits. If they are, it would be wise to see a professional to help you address this. You can run a full iron panel, a complete blood count (CBC), a GGT (gamma-glutamyl transferase) test, and a metabolic panel. The GGT test measures your blood's level of GGT, an enzyme primarily found in the liver that helps metabolize drugs and other toxins. Excessive iron accumulation in the body can damage the liver, and as the liver is damaged, it releases more GGT into the bloodstream. It's also helpful to measure your copper and ceruloplasmin levels as these can be affected by iron overload as well.

This is a particularly important issue for me as I was born with thalassemia, a genetic form of anemia. A screening test at the University of Illinois Medical Center diagnosed me with this problem while I was overseeing the Kidney Transplant Preservation Lab there. It was the job I had before medical school. After I graduated and started practicing, I diagnosed my dad with this anemia. We began regular blood donations for him, and I believe that added twenty years to his life. He passed away at eighty-nine on no medications.

There are several strategies you can use to keep your iron in check. First, you can inhibit iron absorption by consuming coffee or tea with your meals. The polyphenols and tannins in these beverages bind to iron, reducing its absorption. I often recommend this simple strategy to patients who need to lower their iron intake but don't want to give up iron-rich foods entirely.

Certain supplements can also help inhibit iron absorption when taken with iron-rich foods. These include curcumin, quercetin, silymarin (an extract from milk thistle), and alpha-lipoic acid. These supplements work by binding to the iron, preventing its absorption.

Silymarin deserves special mention, especially for those with hemochromatosis. There are different types of hemochromatosis. The most common is hereditary hemochromatosis, caused by a mutation in the HFE gene. There's also secondary hemochromatosis, which results from conditions that cause excess iron in the body. Silymarin can help in managing these conditions by lowering iron levels as well as protecting and repairing the liver.

By prioritizing protein and adding collagen to your diet, you are not just feeding your body—you're nourishing it at the cellular level. You're supporting its processes and defenses against age-related decline.

I've seen patients adopt these principles to transform their health, leaving them feeling more vital and alive than they have in years. It's about giving your body the tools it needs to thrive, not just survive.

CHAPTER 10

Your Gut's Rainbow: A Simple Introduction to Carb-Fueled Gut Repair

Achieving optimal metabolism hinges on your ability to burn carbohydrates properly. When it comes to carbs, there are two very different viewpoints. Some argue that since your body can produce carbohydrates on its own, they must be nonessential nutrients. Others believe that the very fact that your body makes carbohydrates is proof that you require them. The latter perspective hits the nail on the head.

While it's true that your body can make carbohydrates, relying on this mechanism alone comes at a huge cost to your health. When you don't consume enough carbs through your diet, your body must work overtime to produce them internally. This process involves raising your stress hormones to break down your muscle tissue or dietary protein to convert it to glucose. Your body is quite literally destroying your muscles, the most metabolically active tissue, just to supply itself with glucose. Hardly a good trade!

Gluconeogenesis is the process of making glucose from noncarbs. It is always happening in the background, to some extent. However, it kicks into high gear when you restrict your carb intake. This is why nutritionists, dietitians, and sports nutrition experts say that "carbs are protein sparing." When you eat carbs, your body can use dietary protein for vital tasks. It doesn't need to use the protein to make carbs because the carbs provide the necessary glucose for your survival.

This chapter will clear up many myths you may have heard about carbs and focus on their benefits. First, we'll talk about how carbs are your body's primary energy source, fueling everything from your brain to your muscles, especially during peak performance. We'll also explore the role of fiber-rich carbs in keeping your digestive system happy and healthy.

Next, we'll break down the different types of carbs: simple and complex. We'll cover examples of each and discuss how they impact your body differently. You'll discover which carbs are best for sustained energy and which ones have some drawbacks. We'll even touch on the relationship between certain carbs and cancer.

We will also review why you need a variety of carb sources in your diet. These include well-cooked veggies, fruits, natural sugars, and starchy carbs. Fiber is another key player in the carb game. We'll explore the differences between soluble and insoluble fiber and see how they affect your digestive health. You will also learn about the link between fiber, gut bacteria, and butyrate, a short-chain fatty acid.

We must also address small intestinal bacterial overgrowth (SIBO) and candida, a common yeast infection, when discussing carbs and gut health. Many believe that removing carbs is the answer for these conditions, but this is untrue. Removing the trigger may suppress your symptoms, but it will not fix the root cause, which is insufficient energy production in your gut.

Finally, we will discuss how to optimize your carb intake, taking your age, sex, activity level, and metabolic rate into consideration. By the end of this chapter, you'll appreciate carbohydrates as crucial for your health, energy, and vitality.

Feeling Drained? Discover How Carbs Fuel Your Brain and Keep You Sharp

Carbohydrates break down into glucose, the main energy source for your cells, especially your brain cells. But the importance of carbohydrates goes beyond providing energy. Carbohydrates also play a key role in maintaining a healthy metabolism. Furthermore, they are essential for supporting a healthy gut microbiome. Because beneficial gut bacteria thrive on the fiber in complex carbs, fiber helps maintain a diverse and balanced gut flora, which is crucial for proper digestion, nutrient absorption, and immune function.

Many parts of your body need carbohydrates to function well. These include your red blood cells, central nervous system, kidneys, eye tissues, and muscles, especially during strength training. Even your brain requires them for optimal performance. These organs can't rely solely on fatty acids or ketones for energy, which is why it's important to maintain a minimum blood glucose concentration to keep these cells fueled.

Your Brain Runs Better on Glucose

You're a busy professional, juggling many projects and deadlines. By day's end, you feel mentally drained. Why? The answer might lie in your brain's favorite fuel source: glucose. Your brain is like a high-powered computer—it never sleeps. It constantly processes information and keeps your body running. But to do this, it needs a steady supply of energy, and that energy comes primarily from carbs. Lack of carbs in your diet may cause brain fog, fatigue, and trouble concentrating.

Your brain might only make up about 2 percent of your body weight, but it's a real energy hog, consuming a whopping 20 percent of your total calories. That's right—one-fifth of all the energy you consume goes straight to your brain. If you don't give your brain the glucose it needs, you could be in serious trouble. I'm not just talking about brain fog—extremely low glucose can cause a hypoglycemic coma. If this happens, your brain cannot support vital functions, like breathing.

You might be thinking, "Can't my brain just use other fuel sources, such as ketones or lactate, when glucose is low?" And you're right; your brain is adaptable. Fasting or low-carb diets can make your liver produce ketones from fats. These can cross the blood-brain barrier and provide up to 60 percent of your brain's energy. Lactate, produced by your muscles and brain cells called astrocytes, can also be used as a brain fuel.

But here's the catch: even with these alternative fuel sources, your brain still needs glucose to function at peak performance levels. This is especially true for the completion of complex tasks. So, while ketones and lactate can help in a pinch, they can't completely replace carbs.

In fact, your brain needs at least 125 grams of carbs per day to keep running smoothly. When you factor in the rest of your body, you are looking at a total minimum adult requirement of 250 grams of carbs per day. If you have nonalcoholic fatty liver disease (NAFLD), which affects 26 to 40 percent of the population, your liver's ability to store glycogen (the storage form of glucose) may be reduced by up to 50 percent. In this case, you may need even more carbs.

If You Struggle at the Gym, Use Carbs to Help You Build Muscle and Recover Faster

Let's shift gears and talk about how carbs fuel your physical performance. If you work out or want to stay active, carbs are your secret weapon. They help build and maintain muscle and boost performance. Whether you're at the gym, running sprints, or simply living an active life, carbs are vital in fueling your muscles and supporting your fitness goals.

Think of your muscles like a high-performance sports car. Just as that car needs premium gas to reach top speeds, your muscles need glycogen to perform at their best. Glycogen is stored in your muscles as well as your liver. Fat is a great fuel for low-intensity activities, but it breaks down too slowly for the intense bursts of energy you need during a workout.

You might be shocked to learn just how quickly your body can burn through its glycogen stores during exercise. A single strength-training session can deplete your muscle glycogen levels by a whopping 24 to 40 percent. Even just three sets of twelve repetitions performed to failure can result in a 26 percent decrease in muscle glycogen. That's a sizable chunk of your energy reserves gone in a short amount of time.

This rapid depletion of glycogen has serious implications for muscle growth and recovery. Studies show that when your glycogen is low, muscle breakdown can more than double compared to when glycogen is full. Eating carbs after your workout signals your body that it should focus on rebuilding and repairing muscle, not breaking it down further.

But the benefits of carbs for muscle growth don't stop there. Eating carbs in your post-workout meal also lowers stress hormones. High cortisol can hinder your muscle growth and recovery. One study found that carbs in a post-workout meal cut cortisol levels by 11 percent. In contrast, the no-carb group saw a 105 percent rise in peak cortisol.

If you engage in strength training and don't eat enough carbs, your body must produce glucose by sacrificing muscle. This is the opposite of what you want when trying to build and maintain muscle mass.

Moreover, a long-term, carb-deprived state can downregulate your metabolism and impair your thyroid function. This leaves you in survival mode. So, if you want to give your body the best possible chance to build and preserve muscle, make sure to include carbs in your diet. Before and/or after workouts, eat a mix of simple and complex carbs. This will replenish your glycogen and support muscle growth.

The key takeaway is that carbs are not your enemy. They are your body's preferred fuel for intense exercise. They are also key to a muscle-building diet. Carbs can help you reach your fitness goals, so use them wisely and you will achieve the strong, healthy body you want. I previously discussed some of the benefits of increased muscle mass, but there are more. When you have more muscle, you burn more fat at rest. Your glucose use and insulin sensitivity improve, which is great news for your health. You might also see benefits to your mental health because there's a strong link between fitness and well-being.

Greater muscle mass increases your metabolism, clears LDL cholesterol, and strengthens your bones. Your body composition improves, you lower your risk of heart disease, and your physical function gets a boost. It's like a domino effect of health benefits.

You might also be surprised to know that carbs support your digestive health. They provide energy for your gut and intestinal cells, and supply micronutrients for converting food to ATP (adenosine triphosphate). Finally, they provide fiber to feed your gut microbiome. The right kinds of carbs play a crucial role in keeping your gut happy and healthy.

Why is gut health so important? Well, as we learned in earlier chapters, it affects just about everything in your body. The state of your gut influences your nutrient absorption, hormone balance, energy levels, and even your mood. It affects systemic inflammation and immune function. It also impacts your risk for neuropsychiatric disorders. In short, a healthy gut is key to your overall health.

Unfortunately, conventional medicine often misses the mark when it comes to gut health. Instead of addressing root causes, many doctors focus on treating symptoms. Got heartburn? Here's an antacid. Irritable bowel syndrome? Try some fiber supplements, laxatives, or even an antidepressant. Food sensitivities? Just avoid those foods. But these approaches don't solve the underlying problems.

How the Right Carbs Can Heal Digestive Issues and Boost Your Overall Health

Many people don't realize that food sensitivities are often secondary problems resulting from digestive issues. In a healthy state, your gut barrier selectively allows digested nutrients to enter your body at the right time. But when your gut barrier is compromised due to low energy production, partially digested food particles can slip through. This causes inflammation that can lead to autoimmune and neurological issues.

So how do we approach improving gut health? It starts with boosting your energy production and metabolism. This might involve removing gut-irritating foods and additives that slow transit time. You might also need to temporarily remove your unique trigger foods to stop the inflammation cycle and give your body the space it needs to heal.

Here's some good news that might surprise you: your body replaces the lining of your gut every three days! This means that those long, drawn-out gut-healing protocols you might have heard about don't really make sense. If you're still trying to fix your gut after several months or even years, it's time to rethink your approach. If you have good energy metabolism, fixing your gut should take a matter of weeks, not months.

Do not fall for the low-carb fads that promise quick fixes but leave you feeling drained and your gut health compromised. Instead, embrace the power of carbs as part of a balanced, nutrient-dense diet. Choose high-quality carbohydrates, and eat them in amounts that suit your activity level and health goals. You are supporting your body's processes, from muscle building to gut repair. This will promote your long-term health and vitality.

How Your Gut Health Hinges on the Right Balance of Bacteria

Let's dive into the fascinating world of fiber and gut health. Fiber, a unique carb that your body cannot digest, is vital for a healthy digestive system. Think of fiber as nature's broom. It sweeps your intestines and keeps everything moving. It's your best friend when it comes to preventing constipation and keeping you regular. Plus, it has this amazing ability to help you feel fuller for longer after meals, which can be a real game changer if you're trying to manage your weight.

Fiber also plays an essential role in preventing the recirculation of toxins and excess hormones. Without enough fiber, 90 to 95 percent of your bile—which contains toxins, mycotoxins, pesticides, and excess hormones—can be recirculated in your body. This process, called enterohepatic recirculation, is something you want to avoid. Fiber is also like a gourmet meal for your beneficial gut bacteria. These little guys love to munch on fiber, producing amazing stuff called short-chain fatty acids (SCFAs). One of the most important SCFAs is butyrate, which is like a superfood for your gut lining. It helps keep your gut strong and healthy, warding off diseases of all kinds.

But here's where things get interesting—we call it the fiber paradox. While fiber is great for your gut, it requires the right balance of gut bacteria to really work its magic. If your gut is out of whack, with too many harmful bacteria and not enough of the good guys, fiber ends up feeding the bad bacteria instead. These harmful bacteria, which I call oxygen-tolerant bacteria, can cause a range of uncomfortable digestive symptoms. They love to ferment fiber, and in doing

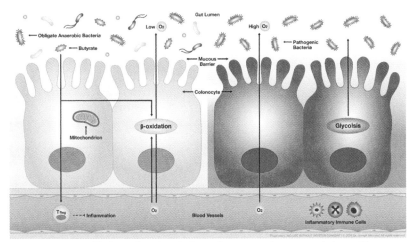

Comparison of balanced and imbalanced gut microbiomes and their effects on colon health. This illustration depicts the stark contrast between a balanced gut microbiome (left) and an imbalanced one (right), highlighting their impacts on colon health and function.

Balanced Gut Microbiome *(left panel). The environment is characterized by low oxygen (O_2) levels, favoring oxygen-intolerant obligate anaerobic bacteria. These beneficial microbes metabolize dietary fiber to produce short-chain fatty acids, such as butyrate. The colonocytes (colon cells) are shown in a healthy state, using beta oxidation for optimal ATP production. This is evidenced by the presence of healthy mitochondria. The mucus barrier is intact, providing protection against pathogens. T regulatory (Treg) cells are present, indicating controlled inflammation. The overall ecosystem supports a well-functioning, healthy gut lining.*

Imbalanced Gut Microbiome *(right panel). A high-oxygen environment is dominated by oxygen-tolerant and pathogenic bacteria. The colonocytes appear inflamed and rely on glycolysis for energy production, a less efficient process resulting in lower ATP levels. The mucus barrier is compromised, allowing closer contact between pathogens and the gut lining. Inflammatory immune cells are present in the underlying tissue, suggesting ongoing inflammation. This environment is conducive to increased endotoxin production and may lead to digestive discomfort when dietary fiber is consumed.*

245

so, they overproduce endotoxins. Remember when we learned that endotoxins are toxic substances bound to the cell walls of bacteria and are released into your system when the cells die? They're bad news for your gut and can really mess with your energy metabolism.

Speaking of energy metabolism, let's talk about what causes poor energy production in your gut. There are three main culprits: linoleic acid (LA), excess estrogen, and electromagnetic fields (EMFs). These factors can hinder the energy production in your gut, making your large intestine "leaky" and allowing in unwanted oxygen. This lets disease-causing bacteria thrive and harms your important beneficial bacteria.

A healthy gut has a balanced microbiome. In an ideal scenario, your gut is dominated by oxygen-intolerant microbes in a low-oxygen environment. An imbalanced gut is dominated by oxygen-tolerant bacteria in a high-oxygen environment, and this imbalance can lead to all sorts of health issues.

The Balancing Act of Fiber to Optimize Your Bacteria and Energy Production

Let's talk more about how your gut cells, specifically your colono-cytes, produce energy. They have two main options: beta oxidation and glycolysis. Beta oxidation is the preferred method, as it is how your cells burn fat for energy and use up oxygen in the process. This helps maintain the low-oxygen environment in which beneficial bacteria thrive. Glycolysis is less efficient. It doesn't use oxygen, which can lead to a high-oxygen environment where harmful bacteria can thrive.

This is where those important short-chain fatty acids come into play again. SCFAs energize your colonocytes and signal the cells to prefer beta oxidation over glycolysis. It's like they're telling your gut cells, "Hey, let's do this the right way!"

What happens when energy production in your gut is low? Well, it can shift your colonocyte metabolism toward glycolysis. This lowers oxygen use and ATP production, shifting your microbial community. The beneficial, oxygen-intolerant bacteria cannot survive in this high-oxygen environment, which means the harmful, oxygen-tolerant bacteria take over. This leads to an imbalance in your gut bacteria and leaky gut, causing food intolerances and endotoxemia—a condition where endotoxins enter your bloodstream.

So, fiber is crucial for a healthy gut. It fuels beneficial bacteria to produce important SCFAs, and your colonocytes need these SCFAs for optimal energy production. A lack of fiber can kill your gut's beneficial bacteria, hindering energy production in your colonocytes and setting off a chain of self-perpetuating gut health issues.

But for those with poor gut health, fiber can end up feeding the bad bacteria and causing negative symptoms. It's important to understand that this is not fiber's fault but rather the current state of your gut. We do not need another food fear in the health and wellness space.

If you're dealing with poor gut health, the first step is not necessarily to add more fiber to your diet. Your gut needs to be primed and ready before you can load up on fiber. Start by eliminating the key culprits damaging your gut—things like vegetable oils and processed foods, all plastic exposures, and EMFs.

Focus on restoring your cellular energy production. As you do this, you'll need to consume carbs. But choose carbs that are extremely low in fiber or even without any fiber at first. This gives your gut a chance to heal and allows your microbial population to come into better balance. Once you have taken these steps, you can slowly begin to add more fiber to feed those SCFA-producing bacteria. It's a process, but it's worth it for the long-term health of your gut.

Choosing the Right Fiber Will Determine If Your Health Is Good or Bad

Someone with good gut health and a strong metabolism does not need to worry about fiber. Eating a variety of healthy foods will meet their fiber needs. But when your gut is in a compromised state, paying attention to the type and quantity of fiber you eat is a foundational step to healing. The goal is to eat enough fiber to form a good stool. It should help rid your body of excess hormones and toxins, but it must not cause constipation or feed harmful bacteria.

If you're dealing with gut issues and you're not quite ready to dive into a high-fiber diet, that's okay. In fact, a low-fiber diet might be exactly what your body needs. To heal your gut, cut fiber for a bit. Focus on easy-to-digest simple sugars. It's like pressing the reset button on your digestive system.

As you start to feel better, slowly reintroduce fiber into your diet. This gradual approach lets oxygen-intolerant bacteria reestablish themselves. Over time, you will be able to tolerate a wider variety of fibrous foods.

One of the most effective fibers for nourishing bacteria is inulin. But use caution. If your gut microbiome is imbalanced, inulin can cause harmful bacteria to grow quickly. This overgrowth can lead to severe health complications and, in extreme cases, may even be life-threatening. You must approach fiber supplementation with caution and expert guidance.

Think of it like this: If you've been injured, you don't immediately jump back into intense exercise. You start with gentle movements and gradually increase the intensity as you heal. The same principle applies to your gut. Start with easily digestible foods and slowly work your way up to more complex, fiber-rich options as your gut heals and becomes stronger.

There's more to the world of fiber and carbohydrates and how they impact your gut health. You might be surprised to learn that not all high-fiber foods are beneficial for everyone. Some popular "health foods"—such as chia, flax, and pumpkin seeds—are high in polyunsaturated fatty acids (PUFAs), which harm gut health.

Flax seeds are also very estrogenic—even more so than soy. In today's world, you are already exposed to plastics, pesticides, and estrogens in your food. You do not need more estrogen receptor activators in your diet. They are a primary mitochondrial poison and will decrease your cellular energy.

When it comes to selecting fiber types, consider your current gut health. If you have a compromised gut, soluble fiber can sit in your gut and putrefy. It's easily fermented by gut bacteria, which can worsen issues like leaky gut and bacterial overgrowth. Insoluble fiber is less likely to be fermented by intestinal bacteria.

When undesirable bacteria ferment soluble fibers, they produce by-products that can harm your gut health, including gases and other substances that cause discomfort. They also inflame the gut, which can damage its lining and worsen leaky gut syndrome and many autoimmune conditions.

A lack of dietary fiber will harm your gut, making it unable to produce short-chain fatty acids like butyrate. This will compromise your gut's protective functions and start a vicious cycle.

Navigating Simple and Complex Carbohydrates to Produce Maximum Energy

Both simple and complex carbs are necessary for good health and play important roles in your physiology. Simple carbs, like those found in fruits and honey, replenish liver glycogen quickly. They help with estrogen detox and converting T4 into the active thyroid hormone T3. Both processes occur in the liver. Simple carbs are also easy for your body to digest, due to their structure. Healthy foods high in simple carbs include ripe fruit, fresh-squeezed fruit juice, raw honey, organic sugar, and maple syrup.

Complex carbs are made of longer, more complex chains of sugar molecules. They take longer to digest than simple carbs and are great for replenishing your muscle glycogen. They also signal abundance and homeostasis to your body. Examples of complex carbs include starches like rice, potatoes, and bread. These complex chains require more energy to digest, so people with poor gut health may not tolerate them as well.

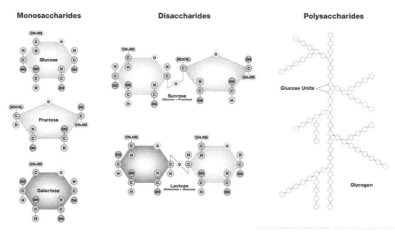

Structural representations of carbohydrates: monosaccharides, disaccharides, and polysaccharides.

Ideally you want to be able to tolerate starchy foods because it's the best fuel for sustained energy. While starches produce similar ATP levels as other glucose carbs, they release glucose for energy more slowly than simple sugars.

However, if your gut is impaired, starches and other fiber-rich foods are problematic as they will feed the pathogenic bacteria in your gut. These bacteria produce endotoxin, which will impair your mitochondria and lower your energy. Hence, you need to incorporate starchy foods slowly.

As your gut recovers, it becomes more friendly to beneficial bacteria. In the early phase of gut healing, low-fiber grains such as white rice can be helpful. They provide a gentle transition. As your gut flora gets more balanced, you can slowly add other starches. Sweet potatoes are a good choice. They support a healthy, diverse microbiome without overloading it.

To clarify, many complex carbs are high in starch and fiber. But some foods can be high or low in either starch or fiber while still being complex carbs. For example, white rice is high in starch but low in fiber, while broccoli is rich in fiber but low in starch. Yet both are complex carbs.

It is possible for someone with poor gut health to tolerate fiber but not starch, or vice versa. This tolerance varies by gut issues and how carbs are processed.

In conditions like small intestinal bacterial overgrowth (SIBO), bacteria overgrow in the small intestine. Starches are often poorly tolerated because they ferment quickly, causing gas and bloating. Fiber, particularly soluble fiber, may be better tolerated as it tends to ferment more slowly. The opposite is often true for those with irritable bowel syndrome (IBS). Some fibers, especially insoluble ones, can worsen symptoms. They add bulk and speed up your digestion. Starches, which break down more easily into sugars, might be better tolerated in this case. Interestingly, simple carbs—often considered empty-calorie junk food—are rapidly absorbed in your small intestine. They never reach your large intestine, where most gut bacteria live. As a result, simple carbs rarely fuel the growth and activity of harmful oxygen-tolerant bacteria that produce endotoxins. In fact, they dramatically reduce endotoxin production by limiting the fermentable substrates that reach your colon.

But before you start loading up on simple carbs, consider the broader context and potential drawbacks of relying on them too heavily. While they may not directly feed certain gut bacteria, a diet high in simple sugars can still negatively affect your health. Excessive intake of simple carbs is linked to insulin resistance, obesity, and a higher risk of chronic diseases, including type 2 diabetes and heart disease.

So, what can you do to support your gut health?

The key is balance and understanding your body. If you have gut issues, you need to seriously limit your complex carbs and focus on simple carbs to help your gut heal. But as your gut health improves, you should aim to include a variety of both simple and complex carbs in your diet.

Remember, everyone's gut is unique. What works for one person may not work for another. Pay attention to how different foods make you feel. Work with a health-care professional who knows gut health when changing your diet.

Switching Gears:
How Increasing Carbs Helped Me Build Muscle and Improve Health

During my low-carb phase, I restricted carbs to fewer than 100 grams per day, far below my requirement of around 400 grams due to my high exercise level. I then gradually increased my intake to 500–600 grams of carbs. Within a few months, I had gained six pounds.

You might think this weight gain was predictable, but a closer look reveals a surprising story. Using a professional lean body mass analyzer to track my body fat percentage, I found that when I started this experiment, my body fat was 11 percent. After gaining weight, it dropped to 5 percent. This suggests that the weight gain was due to increased muscle, not fat.

Moreover, my fasting insulin dropped to 1.4, and my HOMA-IR insulin resistance score was 0.2, which is exceptionally low. In my case, increasing carbs clearly moved my health markers in a positive direction.

Carbs Made Simple: A Color-Coded System to Guide Your Gut Health Journey

Let's explore a new way to eat carbs. It might change your health journey for the better. I know what you're thinking: "But, Dr. Mercola, haven't we always been told to focus on complex carbs?" Well, hold on to your hats because we're about to challenge that conventional wisdom.

Here's the deal: we're going to temporarily rank simple carbs over complex ones. Before you dismiss this idea, hear me out. The goal here is twofold: to support your mitochondrial energy production and promote gut healing. Think of it as a strategic reset for your body.

Why does this approach work?

Simple carbs provide a quick energy boost for your cells and mitochondria. It's like giving your body's energy factories an immediate fuel injection. At the same time, this approach gives your gut a chance to rest and heal. A compromised digestive system can worsen your symptoms. That's because fiber and prebiotics in complex carbs feed oxygen-tolerant gut bacteria. By cutting complex carbs and focusing on simple, digestible ones, you're giving your gut a much-needed break.

Here's how to implement this approach.

For those of you dealing with severely compromised gut health, start with pure sugar water. I can almost hear the gasps of horror, but trust me, this is a temporary measure to jump-start your healing process. The key is to sip it slowly over time. Never drink more than an ounce at a time or you run the risk of metabolic disburbances by spiking your insulin.

During this initial phase, you could put one-half pound, up to a full pound, of pure dextrose (glucose) into a half gallon of water and sip it slowly all day. Once your gut health has improved, you can switch your primary carb source to whole foods. More than likely, you'll also need to eat more frequently than you're used to during this transition to avoid hypoglycemia. Eating every three to four hours, with snacks throughout the day, is crucial when relying on simple carbs for energy.

As your mitochondrial energy production continues to improve and your gut starts to heal, you will begin the transition back to complex carbs. This is a slow and steady process—don't rush it. Your body needs time to adapt to the fermentable fibers and prebiotics in whole grains, legumes, and vegetables. It must build a tolerance to them.

Once you're able to include more complex carbohydrates in your diet, you'll start to notice significant benefits. You'll be able to extend the time between meals to between four and six hours, and many people find they can comfortably switch to a three-meals-a-day approach. This is because complex carbs digest more slowly, providing a steady stream of energy.

The following chart breaks down several types of carbohydrate sources and how they fit into this plan. We can categorize them into three groups: green, yellow, and red.

CARBOHYDRATE SOURCES

Green	Yellow	Red
Dextrose	Maple Syrup	Non-Starchy Veggies
	Fruit Juice with Pulp	
White Rice	Whole Fruits	Starchy Veggies
	Custom Pasta	Beans and Legumes
Sucrose	Pulp-Free Fruit Juice	
	Root Veggies	Whole Grains

Classification of carbohydrate sources. This color-coded chart illustrates a strategic progression of carbohydrate sources, designed to support the rehabilitation of gut health and optimize energy production. The categorization is based on the complexity and digestibility of the carbohydrates.

In the green category, we have dextrose, white rice, and sucrose. We're going to focus on these carbs initially because they are easily digestible and provide quick energy without overtaxing your compromised digestive system.

The yellow category, the next step in our progression, includes maple syrup, fruit juice with and without pulp, whole fruits, and root vegetables. They offer more nutrients and fiber than the green category but are still relatively easy on the digestive system.

Finally, we have the red category, the most complex carbs: non-starchy veggies, starchy veggies, beans and legumes, and whole grains. They offer many health benefits but can be challenging for a compromised gut to handle.

The Carbohydrate Spectrum: From Simple Sugars to Complex Starches

Let's explore the fascinating world of carbohydrates. We'll look at their forms and how they affect your body. We'll start with the simplest and work our way up to more complex carbs, each playing a unique role in your health and energy levels.

Level 1: Dextrose/Glucose—the Simplest Sugar

At the top of our carbohydrate hierarchy sits dextrose, also known as glucose. This is the simplest form of sugar, with a glycemic index (GI) of 100—the highest on the scale. Dextrose is essentially pure energy in its most accessible form. It contains no fiber and is absorbed directly into your bloodstream, causing rapid spikes in blood sugar levels.

You might be thinking, "Dr. Mercola, isn't this exactly what we're trying to avoid?" Well, not necessarily. In some cases, especially with poor gut health, dextrose can help dramatically and wake up your brain in hours. It is absorbed in your upper colon and very little reaches your large intestine, where disease-causing bacteria live, so it's less likely to cause fermentation or bacterial overgrowth.

However, dextrose should be used cautiously and only temporarily. It's not a long-term solution. After one to two weeks, you should start transitioning to other carb sources. The goal is to heal your body, then shift to a sustainable, whole-food diet.

Level 2: White Rice—the Versatile Grain

White rice is a staple for billions of people worldwide, and for good reason. It has a high GI (70–89) and is easily digestible due to its simple starch structure. Consisting only of dextrose, no fructose, and low fiber content, white rice is a quick source of energy, but it can also lead to rapid spikes in blood sugar levels.

The processing of white rice removes the bran and germ, which eliminates many nutrients. However, this same process makes it easier to digest and can be beneficial for those with compromised gut health. Ideally, choose organic versions that are low in arsenic.

Here's a pro tip: Soak your white rice overnight, then thoroughly rinse it before cooking. This simple step can help remove any impurities. Even better, try cooking your rice in bone broth instead of water. This will add flavor and boost its nutrition. The broth has minerals and amino acids that support metabolism.

Level 3: Sucrose and Table Sugar—the Everyday Sweet Stuff

Moving down our list, we come to sucrose, or table sugar. This is what most people think of when they hear "sugar." It has a moderate GI of 58–65, which means it causes a more gradual increase in blood sugar compared to dextrose. Like dextrose, sucrose contains no fiber and is easily digested and absorbed.

Sucrose is a disaccharide, meaning it's made up of two simple sugar molecules: glucose and fructose. The fructose is why sucrose is below dextrose and white rice in the table. While sucrose is low in micronutrients, it can be a useful transitional carb source as you move away from dextrose.

As with dextrose, it's best to dissolve sucrose in water and sip it slowly to avoid rapid blood sugar spikes. And again, this is not a long-term solution but rather a stepping stone in your journey back to health.

Level 4: Maple Syrup—Nature's Sweet Secret

Maple syrup is often overlooked in discussions about carbohydrates, but it deserves our attention. It has a moderate GI of 54, and releases sugar into the bloodstream more slowly than higher GI sweeteners. Because it contains no fiber, it's also easily digestible.

But here's where maple syrup shines: it's a good source of manganese, providing about 65 percent of your daily requirement in just two tablespoons. Manganese plays a crucial role in bone health, wound healing, and metabolism. Maple syrup also contains small amounts of zinc and other minerals.

When choosing between maple syrup and honey, I recommend maple syrup. It contains no free fructose, and most people find it more palatable. Make sure you're getting the real deal, not maple-flavored corn syrup. Many supermarkets sell artificially flavored corn syrup as maple syrup, so don't be fooled!

Level 5: Fruit Juices with Pulp—a Step Closer to Whole Fruits
Fruit juices with pulp are a step up from their pulp-free counterparts. They have a moderate-to-high GI (50–70) and contain low to moderate amounts of fiber, which slow digestion and absorption, improving control over blood sugar spikes.

These juices keep more of the fruit's original nutrients than strained juices. They're a good source of vitamins (particularly vitamin C), minerals, and some fiber from the pulp. However, the concentration of nutrients is lower than in whole fruits due to processing and dilution.

Pulp-containing fruit juices are more nutritious than pulp-free ones, but they are still more sugary than whole fruits. They should be consumed in moderation within a balanced diet.

Level 6: Whole Fruits—Nature's Perfect Package
Now we're getting to the good stuff. Whole fruits are nature's perfect package of carbs, fiber, and nutrients. They have a low-to-moderate GI (30–60) due to their fiber and natural sugars. This fiber not only slows down sugar absorption but also feeds beneficial gut bacteria.

Fruits are packed with vitamins, minerals, and antioxidants, making them nutritional powerhouses. They're rich in vitamin C, vitamin A, folate, potassium, and magnesium, among others. They also contain various beneficial antioxidants and phytonutrients.

Your primary goal should be to improve your gut health to the point where you can tolerate whole fruits comfortably. Once you reach this stage, you're well on your way to restoring your energy and health. Remember, fruits are not just apples and oranges. Kabocha, butternut, acorn, delicata, and spaghetti squashes are also considered fruits. These should be cooked (roasted or boiled) and can be an excellent and delicious carb source in a balanced diet.

Level 7: Pulp-Free Fruit Juices—Nature's Energy Drink

Next up, we have pulp-free fruit juices. These have a high GI, typically 70–90, and contain extremely low amounts of fiber. They provide quick energy spikes but also lead to rapid drops in energy if consumed in substantial amounts. This is why it is very important to sip fruit juices very slowly. Otherwise you will cause a metabolic imbalance and disturb your insulin levels.

The benefit of pulp-free fruit juices is that they offer more micronutrients compared to pure sugar. They contain vitamins and minerals, particularly vitamin C and potassium. But removing the pulp eliminates most of the fiber and some nutrients bound to it, including certain antioxidants and phytonutrients.

For those with compromised gut health, pulp-free juices can be a good transition from pure sugar solutions to whole fruits. They're easy to digest and provide quick energy, but they introduce some of the beneficial compounds in whole foods. However, it's important to use these juices judiciously. If you rely on pulp-free fruit juices for carbs, you may need to eat more often to avoid low blood sugar.

The reason pulp-free fruit juice is not listed directly below dextrose water is because of its lack of fiber and high-fructose content. When consumed rapidly, fructose will send your insulin level soaring. So, if used, pulp-free juice must be sipped over longer periods of time, just like dextrose water. If you can tolerate it, whole fruit would be a better alternative than pulp-free juice. Whole fruits are among the best carbs you can eat—until you can tolerate starch, such as white rice and sweet potatoes, which is the ultimate fuel.

Level 8: Root Vegetables—the Underground Powerhouses

Root vegetables like carrots, beets, and turnips are often overlooked in talks about carbs, but they're nutritional gems. They have a moderate-to-high GI (50–85), depending on the specific vegetable and how it's prepared. For instance, a raw carrot has a lower GI than a cooked one.

These veggies provide a moderate amount of fiber, which helps regulate digestion and blood sugar levels. They're particularly rich in vitamins A and C, potassium, and antioxidants. The fiber content in root vegetables helps to moderate the digestion of starches and sugars contained within them.

The starch structure of many root vegetables contains a mix of amylose and amylopectin, but the proportion varies. For example, potatoes have more amylopectin, which makes them easier to digest. Carrots and parsnips have less starch but more sugar and fiber.

While root vegetables are nutritious, they do not provide a lot of energy in the form of carbohydrates. They should be part of your diet but not your main carb source if you want to boost your energy levels.

Level 9: Starchy Vegetables—the Energy-Rich Veggies

At the top of our vegetable hierarchy we have starchy vegetables such as potatoes, sweet potatoes, and corn. These have a moderate-to-high GI (55–85), providing a significant energy boost. But don't let that scare you off. These veggies also offer a decent amount of fiber, especially if you eat the skins (where applicable), which moderates the blood sugar response.

Starchy vegetables are nutritional powerhouses. Potatoes, for instance, are excellent sources of vitamin C, vitamin B6, and potassium. Sweet potatoes are high in beta-carotene, which your body converts to vitamin A. These veggies are key to a balanced diet. They are especially important for those limiting grains or other carb sources.

Most starchy vegetables have a lot of amylopectin, a branched starch that is easier to digest than amylose. This results in quicker digestion and absorption, which explains their higher glycemic index. However, the cooking method can influence their digestibility and glycemic impact. Boiling, roasting, or mashing breaks down the starches, which may increase their glycemic impact.

Level 10: Nonstarchy Vegetables

Nonstarchy vegetables are nutritional powerhouses that should form the foundation of your diet. These include leafy greens, cruciferous vegetables, bell peppers, asparagus, cucumbers, mushrooms, and onions. With a low GI of 10–35, they raise blood sugar only a little, making them great for weight management and health.

What sets nonstarchy vegetables apart is their high fiber content. This fiber not only aids digestion but also helps you feel full and satisfied. Plus, it feeds the beneficial bacteria in your gut, supporting a healthy microbiome.

Nonstarchy vegetables are packed with an impressive array of micronutrients. They're bursting with vitamins A, C, K, and various B vitamins, as well as minerals such as iron, calcium, and potassium. These nutrients are essential for everything from immune function to bone health. And the best part? You get all this nutritional goodness for very few calories.

Nonstarchy vegetables are beneficial, but they are not a good source of carbohydrates. Your body needs carbs for energy, so do not rely solely on these veggies to meet your carb needs. Instead, think of them as the supporting cast in your meals—important but not your main energy source.

Lastly, if you're dealing with gut issues, you might need to be cautious with raw vegetables initially. Cooking them makes them easier to digest while still preserving most of their nutritional benefits. As your gut health improves, you can gradually increase your intake of raw veggies.

Level 11: Beans and Legumes

Beans and legumes are often touted as nutritional superstars, and for good reason. They have a low-to-moderate GI (20–50), and provide steady, sustained energy without spiking your blood sugar. This makes them an excellent choice for maintaining stable energy levels throughout the day.

One of the standout features of beans and legumes is their incredibly high fiber content. A single serving can provide 6–10 grams of fiber—a sizable chunk of your daily needs. This fiber, vital for digestion, helps prevent constipation and feeds your good gut bacteria.

But there's a catch. Beans and legumes contain raffinose, a complex carbohydrate that can be challenging for your body to break down, which is why some people experience gas or bloating after eating beans. If you have a compromised gut, limit your intake of beans and legumes until your digestive system heals.

When it comes to micronutrients, beans and legumes are packed with B vitamins, iron, magnesium, potassium, and zinc. They also provide a good amount of plant-based protein, making them a valuable addition to vegetarian and vegan diets.

If you include beans and legumes in your diet, choose varieties low in PUFAs and phytoestrogens. My top picks include lentils, kidney beans, cannellini beans, navy beans, black beans, black-eyed peas, and pinto beans. Limit your intake of soybeans and chickpeas due to their higher PUFA and phytoestrogen content.

Level 12: Whole Grains

Whole grains have been a staple in human diets for thousands of years. When prepared properly, they can be an excellent source of nutrition. They usually have a moderate-to-high GI (40–70), so they raise blood sugar more than nonstarchy vegetables or legumes. However, their high fiber content helps to slow down this sugar release, providing more sustained energy.

Whole grains are a fantastic source of fiber. A serving can provide 6–8 grams of fiber, which is important for digestive health, blood sugar control, and a healthy gut microbiome. This fiber content is one of the key differences between whole grains and refined grains such as white flour.

Whole grains are also rich in micronutrients. They're packed with B vitamins, iron, magnesium, and selenium. By keeping the bran, germ, and endosperm intact, whole grains keep all their natural nutritional goodness, which is why they're considered more nutritious than their refined counterparts.

While whole grains can be beneficial, they're not for everyone. If you have a compromised gut or are dealing with certain health issues, you might need to limit or avoid grains, at least temporarily. Many grains have antinutrients like lectins and oxalates that can block nutrient absorption and may upset sensitive stomachs.

When it comes to preparing whole grains, proper cooking methods are key. Soaking, sprouting, and pressure-cooking brown rice will boost digestibility and nutrients. Oatmeal should be well cooked, and be sure to avoid those trendy overnight oats as raw oats can be harder on your digestive system.

Pasta, while a popular staple, cannot be tolerated by many. If you want to add pasta to your diet, carefully consider the flour it's made from. If made with wheat, the wheat flour needs to be organic, non-GMO certified, not brominated, and not fortified with iron. Wheat flour used to make sourdough bread should also meet these qualifications. If your gut health is poor, white rice pasta is a safer option. Another alternative would be to use spaghetti squash or sweet potatoes, cut with a handheld spiralizer.

Understanding this carb spectrum is key to a better diet. It's vital if you have gut issues or want more energy. Listen to your body. If needed, start with easily digestible carbs and gradually introduce more complex, nutrient-dense options as your gut health improves.

Your journey to optimal health is unique, and it may require unconventional approaches like this one. Trust the process, be patient with your body, and look forward to the vibrant health that awaits you once you've healed. And remember, this information is a guide. It's necessary to work with a health-care professional who tailors advice to your needs and health.

Sourdough Bread Benefits

Sourdough bread has been making a comeback in recent years. Unlike modern bread, which uses packaged yeast, sourdough bread is leavened with wild yeasts and bacteria in a sourdough starter. This natural fermentation process brings some impressive benefits to the table.

First, sourdough fermentation significantly reduces the amount of fermentable carbohydrates and free glucose in the bread. This means it's easier on your digestive system and less likely to cause rapid spikes in your blood sugar. It's like getting the comfort of bread without the usual carb crash.

Second, the fermentation process breaks down starches and gluten, which makes it more digestible than regular bread. In fact, studies have shown that sourdough bread is about 16 percent more digestible than bread made with baker's yeast. The protein in sourdough bread also has a higher biological value, meaning your body can use it more efficiently.

Third, sourdough bread has less gluten than regular bread. Surprising, right? The lactobacilli in the sourdough starter begin to break down the gluten in the flour during fermentation. This is why many people who have trouble with regular bread find that they can tolerate sourdough.

Lastly, sourdough has more nutrients and better nutrient absorption than regular bread. The fermentation process can increase the levels of certain nutrients and make others more accessible to your body. It's like unlocking the nutritional potential of the grains.

Nixtamalized Corn Benefits

Nixtamalization is a fascinating traditional food preparation method. This ancient process involves soaking dried corn kernels in a solution of calcium hydroxide (lime) and water. The resulting corn flour, known as masa harina, offers some impressive nutritional benefits.

A key benefit of nixtamalization is a big boost in bioavailable vitamin B3 (niacin). In untreated corn, niacin is bound to starches and can't be absorbed by your body. Even the acidic environment of your stomach can't release it. But the alkali treatment of nixtamalization makes this niacin bioavailable, meaning your body can use it.

Nixtamalization also boosts the calcium content of corn products. According to Amanda Gálvez, PhD, a food science professor at the National Autonomous University of Mexico in Mexico City, nixtamalized corn contains thirteen times more calcium than untreated corn. The high calcium content, plus corn's natural phosphorus, creates a better calcium-to-phosphorus ratio. It is key for nutrient absorption.

Nixtamalization also significantly reduces the phytic acid content in corn. Phytic acid is an antinutrient that interferes with the absorption of minerals like iron and zinc. By reducing phytic acid, nixtamalization increases the nutrient bioavailability of corn.

Here's another impressive feat: nixtamalization can reduce mycotoxin levels by up to 90 percent. Mycotoxins are toxic compounds produced by certain molds that grow on crops. By reducing these, nixtamalization makes corn safer to consume.

Lastly, nixtamalization breaks down some of corn's complex starches. This means your body can more easily access and use the nutrients in the corn. It's like predigesting the corn for you!

Importance of Organic Whole Grains

Conventional farming practices often involve heavy use of pesticides and herbicides, including glyphosate. These chemicals can leave residues on the grains, which end up in your body when you consume them.

Glyphosate contamination is a particular concern with oats and wheat. In conventional agriculture, it's common to spray these crops with glyphosate just before harvest. This kills the crops early, pushing the harvest sooner. While this might be convenient for farmers, it's destructive to health.

Corn is another grain where organic sourcing is crucial. Conventionally grown corn is often genetically modified and heavily sprayed with pesticides.

By choosing organic oats, wheat, and corn, you can avoid most contamination problems.

How to Heal Your Gut Without Cutting Carbs and Resolve SIBO

Small intestinal bacterial overgrowth (SIBO) is an often-overlooked condition that can wreak havoc on your digestive system. It occurs when there are too many bacteria in your small intestine. This overgrowth is usually caused by poor gut motility, which means food moves too slowly through your digestive tract.

When you're dealing with SIBO, you might experience a wide range of uncomfortable symptoms, including chronic diarrhea, constipation, bloating, abdominal pain, nausea, acid reflux, and excessive gas. SIBO also causes food sensitivities, like lactose intolerance. Many conventional treatments for SIBO focus on removing carbohydrates from your diet. While this approach might provide short-term relief, it's not a long-term solution. In fact, cutting carbs too much can slow your metabolism, which can worsen the problem. Your body needs carbs for energy, and your gut bacteria need them, too. Starving yourself of carbs isn't the answer.

It's important to understand that SIBO, like many other health issues, stems from a low-energy state in your body. A sluggish metabolism harms your defenses against bacterial overgrowth. These defenses include stomach acid, gut motility, and a working ileocecal valve, which separates your small and large intestines.

Trying to outsmart bacteria by depriving them of nutrients is a losing battle. These microscopic organisms can double their population every twelve hours. Starving them creates an environment where only the toughest bacteria survive. It is evolution in action, and nature always finds a way to adapt and overcome.

If removing carbs isn't the answer, what is? The key to resolving SIBO lies in improving your metabolic rate, supporting thyroid health, and lowering stress levels. These factors all contribute to creating a healthier internal gut environment. It's not just about killing bacteria but also creating an environment where beneficial bacteria thrive and harmful ones cannot.

Addressing SIBO effectively requires a dual approach. First, you need to temporarily eliminate trigger foods that cause discomfort. Second, you need to boost your metabolic rate in order to increase energy and improve digestion, which reduces gas. To do this, fine-tune your diet. Identify which carbs minimize your symptoms.

With SIBO, some dietary fibers can cause digestive issues. They fuel the bacteria in your small intestine. Your initial goal should be to select foods that have less fiber, thereby reducing fuel for bacterial growth. If certain foods are currently causing discomfort, it's wise to avoid them temporarily. The carb classification system I introduced earlier is a great guide for these dietary choices. (See page 253). The best carb for this strategy is dextrose water. It has no fiber and provides a simple way to address the issue. As your tolerance improves, shift to healthier complex carbs.

It's important to remember that healing takes time. Be patient with your body and listen to its signals. As you put these strategies in place, you should notice improvements in your digestive symptoms.

Don't be discouraged if progress seems slow—you're addressing the root cause of the problem, not just masking symptoms.

Overcoming Candida Naturally: The Key to Restoring Your Gut Health

Candida overgrowth is another common gut issue that is often intertwined with SIBO. *Candida albicans* is a type of yeast that naturally exists in your body. It lives in your mucous membranes and, under normal circumstances, coexists peacefully with other gut microbes.

But when the delicate balance of your gut microbiome is disrupted, candida can become problematic. It can colonize your gut, leading to inflammation that triggers a host of digestive issues, including irritable bowel syndrome and leaky gut, as well as more serious conditions such as celiac disease, Crohn's disease, and gastrointestinal cancers.

What makes candida particularly tricky to deal with is its survival tactics when deprived of carbohydrates. When glucose levels are low, candida undergoes a remarkable transformation. It develops invasive filaments that penetrate cell barriers in search of sugar—a dangerous shift from simple yeast cells to a more aggressive form. This ability to adapt not only helps candida survive in hostile environments but also enhances its invasiveness, making it a formidable pathogen. It's another reason why starving problematic microorganisms by cutting carbs will not work long term. Instead, we need to focus on creating an internal environment that keeps candida in check naturally.

Four key factors contribute to candida overgrowth. First is low body temperature. You might not realize it, but fungi thrive when your body temperature drops. It's well documented that higher body temperatures help keep fungal pathogens in check. When your body temperature is low, you're creating a cozy environment for candida to flourish. Ideally you want to maintain a body temperature of 98.6°F to ward off these unwanted guests.

Next, we have elevated levels of estrogen, also known as estrogen dominance. This is a big problem in our modern world where environmental factors and lifestyle choices often lead to estrogen overload. Candida absolutely loves a high-estrogen environment. In fact, studies show that when estrogen levels are low, your cells have a natural resistance to candida. But introduce high levels of estrogen and candida becomes aggressive and invasive. One study even found that high estrogen made candida 8.6 times more invasive!

Low thyroid function is another major player in candida overgrowth. Your thyroid gland helps regulate immune antibodies like IgA. These antibodies protect against pathogens, including candida. Low thyroid function reduces protective antibodies, which makes you more vulnerable to candida.

Lastly, excess iron fuels candida growth. Many people have excess iron stored in their bodies due to fortified foods, multivitamins, and supplements. And stress can disrupt your body's ability to recycle iron. This creates an ideal environment for candida to grow and spread. Research has shown that drugs that lower iron levels can reduce candida survival rates.

The approach to treating candida is remarkably like treating SIBO. It's not about targeting overgrowth but rather creating an environment where candida can't thrive.

The key is to focus on optimizing your metabolism. When your metabolism is functioning well, it naturally keeps candida in check. This means paying attention to your nutrition and lifestyle choices. You need to support your body's energy production to maintain the proper function of your digestive tract.

To guide your dietary choices, use the carb classification system I outlined earlier in this chapter. (See page 253). This system helps you choose carbs that support your metabolism without feeding candida. As with SIBO, dextrose water is an optimal choice to start with. As your body adapts and your tolerance improves, you can slowly switch to healthier complex carbs. These are categorized at higher levels in the carb classification system, and a gradual transition allows your body to heal while still getting the nutrients it needs.

In severe cases, especially in AIDS patients, oral dextrose might not be absorbed quickly enough due to a weak immune system. In these situations, intravenous dextrose can be a lifesaver. It delivers fuel directly to your body and brain, which helps to counteract the problem by bypassing the gastrointestinal tract.

Nourish Your Gut with Simple Cooking Techniques That Make a Big Difference

Cooking methods are a practical way to support your gut-healing journey. How you prepare your food can affect your digestion, especially for a weak digestive system.

When you're dealing with gut issues, raw or lightly cooked foods are challenging for your body to handle. The tough cell walls of plants and complex structures of proteins can be particularly difficult for a weakened gut to break down. But here's where the magic of cooking comes in.

Applying heat and pressure to your food does wonders for digestibility. The cooking process helps break down tough fibers and proteins, making them much easier for your body to handle. It's like giving your digestive system a helping hand, allowing it to extract maximum nutrition from your food with minimal effort.

But who has time to slave over a stove all day? That's where modern kitchen appliances come to the rescue. Electric pressure cookers, such as Instant Pot, are absolute game changers when it comes to gut-friendly cooking. These devices use high pressure to cook food quickly while still breaking down those tough fibers and proteins.

Just be sure to avoid nonstick coatings as they release dangerous fluoride into your kitchen. I use my electric pressure cooker every day—sometimes three times a day—as I prepare meals for myself and my two Great Pyrenees dogs, Joy and Grace.

Imagine a hearty stew or a nourishing soup, packed with tender meats and soft, easily digestible vegetables. With an electric pressure cooker, you get a delicious, gut-friendly meal on the table in a fraction of the time it would take using conventional methods. And the best part? You're not compromising on nutrition. In fact, pressure-cooking can enhance the nutrient availability of your food.

These cooking methods are particularly beneficial if you're dealing with a sensitive gut. They let you try a wider variety of foods, including tougher cuts of meat and fibrous vegetables that might otherwise be off-limits. It's like having a personal chef and a digestive aid all rolled into one!

But the benefits of cooking your own food go beyond the practical aspects. There is something deeply nourishing about the act of preparing a meal from scratch. It's a chance to slow down, connect with your food, and infuse your meals with intention. When you're on a journey to heal your gut, this mindfulness about your self-care can be just as important as the nutrients you're consuming.

So, as you navigate your gut-healing journey, don't underestimate the power of proper food preparation. Embrace these cooking methods as tools in your healing arsenal. They'll not only make your meals more digestible but also more enjoyable and diverse.

Trust Your Gut: How Listening to Your Body Leads to Better Health

To recap, improving your gut health is not a quick fix or a one-size-fits-all solution. Think of it as a marathon, not a sprint. You're in this for the long haul, and small, consistent steps will get you further than drastic, unsustainable changes.

Start by paying attention to how different foods make you feel. Keep a food diary if it helps. Note which foods cause discomfort and which ones make you feel energized and healthy. This information is invaluable as you work to improve your gut health. Remember, you're the expert on your own body. Trust your gut (pun intended) and don't be afraid to adjust your approach based on how you feel.

As you navigate this journey, be kind to yourself. Healing takes time, and there might be setbacks along the way. That's okay. Every step forward, no matter how small, is progress. Celebrate these small victories. Did you introduce a new vegetable without any digestive issues? That's a win! Were you able to enjoy a meal without bloating or discomfort? Celebrate it!

It's also important to manage your stress levels. Stress can have a significant impact on your gut health. Find ways to relax and unwind that work for you, whether it's meditation, yoga, reading, or simply taking a walk in nature. Remember, the goal isn't perfection. It's progress. You're working toward better health, not a perfect diet. There will be days when you indulge in foods that might not be the best for your gut. Don't beat yourself up over it. Just get back on track with your next meal.

As you continue this journey, you might find that your tastes and preferences change. Foods that you once craved may lose their appeal, while foods that you previously disliked become new favorites. This is a normal part of the process as your body adjusts to a healthier way of eating.

And don't be afraid to seek out community. Whether it's a health-care professional, a support group, or friends and family, having a support system makes an enormous difference. Share your successes, challenges, and questions. You might be surprised at how many people are on a similar journey and can offer encouragement and advice.

CHAPTER 11

Embrace Seven Supplement Solutions to Restore Your Mitochondrial Health

Ideally you want most of your day-to-day nutrition to come from real, whole foods. However, in your quest to improve your health, some supplements can provide invaluable support by boosting cellular health as well as your body's ability to recover from daily stress.

Think of supplements as temporary aids, like using a crutch or brace when recovering from a sports injury. They're not meant to be lifelong dependencies but rather stepping stones that guide you back to a state of balance and vitality.

As we talk through each of these super supplements, you'll gain insight into how each one supports your body's natural healing processes and can help you become healthier and more energetic.

Akkermansia: A Keystone Species for Gut Health

Let's start with a true gut health hero: *Akkermansia muciniphila*. You may never have heard of this organism as it was discovered only twenty years ago. As we discussed in previous chapters, this beneficial bacterium is not just a part of your microbiome but a vital guardian of your gut health. It maintains the balance and integrity of your digestive system. It helps your gut's defenses, aids nutrient absorption, and reduces inflammation. So, it's no wonder that *Akkermansia* is the next-generation probiotic supplement. It helps with a surprising range of conditions, including obesity, inflammatory bowel disease, metabolic diseases, and neuropsychiatric disorders.

In an ideal world, *Akkermansia* should make up at least 3–4 percent of a healthy microbiome, and some experts believe that number should be as high as 10 percent. But the reality is quite different. Labs analyzing human microbiome composition suggest that about one-third of people have few to no *Akkermansia* at all. I suspect the main cause of this alarming deficiency is decreased cellular energy that allows oxygen levels to rise in your large intestine, killing *Akkermansia* and other beneficial microbes.

Why is *Akkermansia* so crucial? It makes short-chain fats like butyrate, propionate, and acetate that feed your gut's endothelial cells. These cells, in turn, produce mucin, a thick, protective gel that lines your gastrointestinal tract. Mucin acts like a bike repair kit, covering many leaky gut holes caused by too many oxygen-tolerant bacteria.

A lack of *Akkermansia* means you don't have enough short-chain fatty acids for your colon cells to make mucin. This makes your gut far more susceptible to inflammation, causing a cascade of health issues including digestive disorders, a weakened immune system, high blood pressure, obesity, and diabetes.

A New and Inexpensive Way to Test How Healthy Your Gut Is

You might be wondering how to determine if you have enough *Akkermansia* in your gut. That's where my pioneering work comes in. I have a new, inexpensive home microbiome test that greatly improves gut health assessment. Unlike traditional tests that can cost $500 or more, our new screening method costs one-tenth that, or about the price of dinner for one adult.

This test doesn't just detect the presence of beneficial, oxygen-intolerant, keystone bacteria. It measures their quantity, too. Our test serves two key purposes: First, it provides an accurate baseline assessment of your gut health. Second, it allows you to track your progress as you begin the program outlined in this book. By making this test accessible and encouraging regular testing, we're empowering you to gain the necessary self-knowledge to control your gut health and well-being.

The affordability of this test makes it possible for most people to test twice a year, the way you might track your vitamin D levels. This frequency lets you confirm if you have low levels of these crucial bacteria. It empowers you to manage your gut health by providing data to guide your efforts and measure your success.

Live versus Dead Probiotics and Why It Matters for Your Gut Health

Let's discuss a key point about *Akkermansia* probiotics. Many overlook the difference between live and dead *Akkermansia*. Unlike some traditional probiotics, *Akkermansia* is an oxygen-intolerant anaerobe. That means *Akkermansia* doesn't have a middle ground. It's either alive and ready to colonize your gut, or it's dead and useless.

Until recently, it was impossible to produce live strains of *Akkermansia* for sale on the open market. As I write this in 2024, there is a company very close to providing live strains of *Akkermansia*. If you download the Mercola Health Coach app, you can find out when they are available and how to purchase them.

But beware—some companies have a clever marketing strategy. They claim to "pasteurize" their *Akkermansia* supplements. Pasteurization may seem like a good thing as it implies safety and quality. But in this case, it means they are killing all the live *Akkermansia* bacteria, and dead *Akkermansia* provides far less gut health benefit. It cannot grow and colonize your gut. The difference between live and dead *Akkermansia* is vital for reaping the full benefits of this remarkable microbe.

Recent breakthroughs in producing and maintaining live *Akkermansia* are truly exciting. For the first time, we can reliably deliver this beneficial bacterium to those who need it most. But, as with any emerging field, it's crucial to be an informed consumer.

It's also worth noting that *Akkermansia* supplementation isn't a one-size-fits-all solution. Many people can benefit from boosting their *Akkermansia* levels. But it's wise to work with a health-care practitioner who can guide you in using this supplement.

Empower Your Gut Health with Live Akkermansia Probiotics

Smart financial management focuses on net gains—what you keep after expenses—not gross income. Similarly, with *Akkermansia* probiotics, the key isn't the millions or billions of bacteria you consume, but how many reach your colon alive and active to provide the most benefit.

It's how many reach your colon alive and active. *Akkermansia* are very sensitive to oxygen. This makes their journey through your digestive system very challenging. These beneficial microbes thrive in an oxygen-free environment, and even a brief exposure to oxygen can be fatal for them. This trait makes the delivery method of *Akkermansia* supplements crucial to their effectiveness.

Understanding this helps you choose the most effective supplement. You want to nurture your gut microbiome with live, active *Akkermansia*, as dead or inactive ones won't do you as much good since they don't reproduce. If you want to use *Akkermansia* supplements, look for ones with advanced, dual-timed release capsules or microencapsulation. These technologies keep *Akkermansia* dormant and protected until it reaches your colon, usually in two to four hours.

To maximize the effectiveness of your *Akkermansia* supplement, take it on an empty stomach, ideally first thing in the morning after an overnight fast. Wait at least one to two hours before eating to cut the transit time allowing the bacteria to reach your colon faster—usually within two hours. This will greatly increase the number of live bacteria that make it to your colon.

Avoid taking probiotics with food as this can extend their transit time to your colon to over eight hours. This will likely kill any bacteria long before they reach your colon. So, be mindful of when and how you take your *Akkermansia* probiotics so you can maximize the benefits of this powerful probiotic.

Vitamin D3 and Its Supporting Players: Vitamin K2 and Magnesium

Vitamins D3, K2, and magnesium are a dynamic trio that work together to boost your bone, heart, and immune health. While sunlight is the ideal source of vitamin D, many people can't get enough sun exposure due to lifestyle or geographic constraints. That's where oral supplements come in. They can't fully duplicate the benefits of natural sunlight, though, so only use them as a last resort.

When supplementing with vitamin D3, it's crucial to balance it with vitamin K2 and magnesium. Having enough K2 prevents inappropriate calcification and supports bone and vascular health.

Magnesium, meanwhile, is essential for converting vitamin D into its active form. Large doses of vitamin D can deplete magnesium, so it's wise to take them together. In fact, you'll need less vitamin D when taken with magnesium. The optimal strategy? Take all three together: vitamin D3, magnesium, and vitamin K2. For the average adult with no sun exposure, aim for about 8,000 units of D3, 400 milligrams of magnesium, and 150–200 micrograms of K2 daily. Remember, individual needs may vary, and I'll talk more about finding your proper magnesium dosage later in this chapter. To fine-tune your supplementation, get your vitamin D levels tested twice a year. Aim for a level between 40 and 80 ng/mL.

Thyroid Health: The Metabolic Maestro

Thyroid hormones are vital to nearly every bodily function. They're key players in converting glucose into ATP, your body's energy currency.

Most adults have subclinical or undiagnosed hypothyroidism, often due to omega-6 fats, plastics, and EMFs. These modern-day villains suppress thyroid function and slow down your metabolic rate.

For optimal thyroid health, you need efficient conversion of T4 to T3 in your liver. Several factors can inhibit this process, including cortisol, estrogen, liver issues, excessive PUFA intake, and even endotoxins. Interestingly, low-carb diets also depress T3 levels, which is what happens during starvation.

To support your thyroid, avoid fluoride, chlorine, and flame-retardant chemicals. Invest in a good water purification system to remove these thyroid-disrupting substances. Also, avoid things that raise cortisol and estrogen levels because they inhibit T4 to T3 conversion, too. If you're still struggling with thyroid issues, consider natural desiccated thyroid supplementation. This bioidentical supplement can help with hypothyroidism and boost your vitality.

When starting natural desiccated thyroid, begin with half a grain. Increase the dose every two weeks until your morning temperature stabilizes at 98°F. Some may need a higher T3:T4 ratio for the best results.

Remember, thyroid supplementation is highly individual. Work with a qualified health-care provider to check your specific needs. Your ideal dosage may vary based on your environment, stress levels, and medical history. Most people won't need more than two grains of thyroid, but your dosage may vary.

Progesterone—Your Shield Against Environmental Estrogens

Today you are bombarded by environmental estrogens, and plastics are a major source of these hormone-disrupting compounds. This exposure has created an urgent need for effective solutions. That's where progesterone comes in. It has strong anti-estrogenic effects which protect against estrogen toxicity in men and women.

Progesterone is typically thought of as a female hormone because it is vital for a woman's natural menstrual cycle and reproductive health. It prepares the endometrium for a possible pregnancy. Without enough progesterone, the endometrium may not develop properly, which can cause implantation problems, infertility, and a higher risk of miscarriage.

But progesterone's benefits extend far beyond female reproductive health. It is vital for the bone density, heart health, and immune function of both genders. Progesterone also helps protect against chronic conditions from prolonged hormonal imbalances; cancer is one of the most serious of these risks.

I believe that most adults can benefit from progesterone supplementation. Why? Because environmental estrogens are practically impossible to avoid. Even if you use glass containers and avoid plastic wraps, some exposure is inevitable. Progesterone offers a way to counteract and even reverse the effects of this constant estrogenic assault on your body.

A January 2024 study in *Environmental Health Perspectives* paints a grim picture of our chemical landscape. The study found 279 estrogenic compounds in consumer products, some of which induce mammary tumors in animals. But that's not all. They found 642 more chemicals that could raise breast cancer risk by stimulating estrogen or progesterone signaling. These aren't obscure chemicals either. We're talking about parabens and phthalates that are widely used in cosmetics and personal care products. It also includes pesticide ingredients such as malathion, atrazine, and triclopyr, which are often used on food crops and in pest-control products.

How does progesterone help you navigate this chemical minefield? Think of it as a traffic cop for your hormones. It keeps estrogen in check, preventing it from disrupting your body's hormonal balance.

One of the primary ways it does this is by decreasing the expression of estrogen receptors, which reduces the number of landing spots for estrogen, weakens estrogen's effects and helps alleviate the symptoms of estrogen dominance, such as mood swings, weight gain, and cancer risk.

But progesterone doesn't stop there. It can also improve liver function and bile secretion, as well as help your liver process and excrete estrogen. It's like giving your body's detox systems a turbo boost.

Additionally, progesterone promotes the conversion of estrogen into less potent forms of estrogen, some of which are more biologically active and powerful than others. This conversion is vital to maintaining a healthy hormonal balance because it prevents the negative effects of high estrogen levels.

Progesterone also shines when it comes to mood and brain function. It influences neurotransmitter pathways positively, improving mental health and emotional stability. Its calming effects on your brain help lower the anxiety and irritability often seen with estrogen dominance. Many of my patients told me they feel more balanced and clearheaded after starting progesterone therapy.

And let's not forget about bone health. Progesterone binds to specific receptors on the surface of osteoblasts, your bone-building cells. This interaction kicks off a series of cellular processes that lead to increased production of bone matrix proteins. The result? Stronger, healthier bones. And because progesterone helps reduce harmful cytokines, it has anti-inflammatory effects, creating a better environment for bone formation overall.

As helpful as progesterone is, it isn't a magic bullet. It's one of many powerful tools for your health. Use it wisely and with other strategies to optimize your cellular energy. Keep in mind that as your health improves, you will slowly make more progesterone on your own. You might even find that one day you don't need supplementation at all.

Synthetic Progestins versus Bioidentical Progesterone
When it comes to hormone therapy, not all progesterone is created equal. The difference between synthetic progestins and bioidentical progesterone is crucial yet often overlooked. While they might seem similar on paper, their effects on your body couldn't be more different.

Bioidentical progesterone, as the name suggests, is identical to your body's hormone. It fits perfectly into your progesterone receptors, like a key into a lock. Synthetic progestins are like trying to force a slightly misshapen key into that same lock. Sure, it might turn, but the results are unpredictable and often harmful.

Natural progesterone is a powerful anti-inflammatory. It supports your heart health, especially your vascular system. Synthetic progestins? They do the opposite, increasing inflammation throughout your body, damaging your lipids, and raising your blood pressure. This isn't theoretical—it's a real, measurable effect that can significantly impact your health over time. The Women's Health Initiative study found that synthetic progestins raise the risk of coronary heart disease in women. That's not a risk I'm willing to take, and I don't think you should either.

One of the most alarming side effects associated with synthetic progestins is the increased incidence of blood clots, raising your risk of dying from a blood clot in your lungs. To put it in perspective, the risks are similar to those from smoking or being inactive. That's a hefty price to pay for hormone "therapy."

Synthetic progestins have also been linked to a higher risk of breast cancer—the very condition many women are trying to prevent. This finding shows that synthetic progestins may affect cell growth in a way that increases your cancer risk. In fact, some research suggests synthetic progestins may be even more detrimental in this regard than estrogen itself.

If you are considering hormone therapy, I cannot stress enough the need for a frank, open talk with your health-care provider about the type of progesterone used in your treatment. This isn't just a matter of preference—it's a decision that can significantly affect your health outcomes. Synthetic progestins may be easier to dose and find, but the risks of blood clots, breast cancer, and heart disease aren't worth it. All the health benefits we've discussed are from natural progesterone, and that's why it's the only type I recommend.

Practical Tips on Using Progesterone

How do you use progesterone? You can easily purchase USP (United States Pharmacopeia) grade online. Once you have that, you merely dissolve the powder in natural vitamin E, then apply it to your gums. That's the best way to use it. If using the liquid form, make sure it comes in a glass bottle to avoid contamination by estrogenic plasticizers.

A word on vitamin E: don't use the synthetic stuff. Look for natural vitamin E labeled as "d-alpha tocopherol," the pure D isomer, which is what your body can use. You'll also want to know all the isomers of tocopherols and tocotrienols. They should be the beta, gamma, and delta types in the effective D isomer.

The best time to take progesterone is thirty minutes before bed. It has an anti-cortisol function and will increase GABA levels, promoting a good night's sleep. Now, here's where things get a bit tricky with regulations. The FDA considers transmucosal use of progesterone on your gums a drug and prohibits companies from recommending this on their labels. But it's perfectly legal for a physician to recommend this off-label use. Remember, progesterone is a natural hormone, not a synthetic drug, and is very safe even in high doses.

For women who still menstruate, timing your progesterone with your cycle is crucial. You'll want to supplement during the luteal phase—that's the period after ovulation and before your next period starts. Avoid supplementing with progesterone during the follicular phase, as it can interfere with your natural hormone fluctuations.

To get this right, you'll need to track your cycle closely. Note the first day of your period, which marks the start of the follicular phase. Ovulation typically occurs around the midpoint of your cycle. For a twenty-eight-day cycle, this would be around day 14. Start progesterone supplementation the day after you confirm ovulation and continue for about fourteen days. Stop when you expect your next period to begin.

For postmenopausal women, this cyclical approach isn't necessary. You can start anytime and continue daily administration for six months before taking a one-week break. This helps maintain hormonal balance without the need to track a menstrual cycle.

Remember, progesterone therapy should be individualized. Your needs may vary based on your personal health status, symptoms, and goals. Always work with a health-care provider who knows bioidentical hormone therapy and can help you create a tailored plan. With the right approach, progesterone can be a powerful health tool for achieving hormonal balance and well-being.

Xenoestrogens: The Silent Hormone Disruptors

In today's world, you're facing a hidden threat to your health that's lurking in plain sight. I'm talking about xenoestrogens—synthetic chemicals that mimic estrogen in your body. These sneaky compounds are everywhere, from the food you eat to the clothes you wear, and they're disrupting your hormonal balance.

Let's break down where you're most likely to encounter these hormone disruptors. First up: your food. Shockingly, microparticles have infiltrated our food chain. Plastic waste ends up in our waterways, where it breaks down into tiny particles. Marine life consumes these particles, so when we eat seafood, we ingest a dose of plastic and its xenoestrogens.

But it's not just seafood. If you're not eating organic, you're likely getting a side of xenoestrogens with your fruits and veggies. Hormone disruptors come from many sources. A major one is agricultural chemicals, especially nonorganic pesticides. These chemicals don't just disappear when you wash your produce; they can be absorbed into the plant itself.

Your personal care routine might also be exposing you to xenoestrogens. Many moisturizers, cosmetics, and skin-care products contain phthalates and parabens, both known endocrine disruptors. These chemicals can be absorbed through your skin, adding to your body's toxic load.

Even your wardrobe could be part of the problem. Synthetic clothing fibers, like polyester and spandex, contain high levels of bisphenol A (BPA) that can be absorbed through your skin. Whenever possible, choose natural fibers like cotton, linen, or wool. These materials not only feel great but also help reduce your exposure to synthetic xenoestrogen. And let's not forget about BPA and its chemical cousins lurking in plastic containers and thermal paper receipts.

So how can you protect yourself from this onslaught of xenoestrogens? It starts with making informed choices. Opt for BPA-free materials whenever possible. For personal care products, read the labels. Choose ones without parabens and phthalates.

Perhaps the most impactful change you can make is in your diet. Choosing organic foods can greatly reduce your exposure to agricultural chemicals that act as xenoestrogens. Organic produce might cost a bit more, but consider it an investment in your long-term health. If paying more for organics is a stretch for your budget, the Environmental Working Group publishes the *Dirty Dozen* and *Clean 15* reports each year on the most and least contaminated fruits and vegetables (available at https://www.ewg.org/). Looking at these reports can help you choose the produce you don't need to pay extra for (*Clean 15*) as well as the fruits and vegetables you should either spend more on for the organic version or avoid altogether (*Dirty Dozen*).

Let me be clear: the health implications of xenoestrogen exposure are serious and far-reaching. These chemicals don't just throw your hormones out of whack; they can lead to full-blown estrogen toxicity.

What does estrogen toxicity look like? For starters, you might notice unexplained weight gain, particularly around your midsection. Mood swings can become more frequent and intense. Many people also experience reproductive issues, from irregular menstrual cycles to fertility problems.

But the deadliest effect of long-term xenoestrogen exposure is a higher risk of estrogen-driven cancers. Breast cancer, ovarian cancer, and prostate cancer have all been linked to excessive estrogen levels in the body. When you consider that many of us are exposed to these chemicals daily, it's no wonder we're seeing a rise in hormone-related health issues.

In my practice, I've seen the devastating effects of xenoestrogen exposure up close. One patient stands out. Carla came to me with a puzzling mix of symptoms: unexplained weight gain, mood swings, and irregular periods. Despite countless tests, her previous doctor found nothing, leaving Carla feeling frustrated and hopeless.

After exploring her lifestyle, we found the culprit: xenoestrogens. She was unknowingly bombarding herself with them. Her skin-care products, diet, and new workout gear all exposed her to these dangerous chemicals. Tragically, by the time we uncovered this, it was too late. A routine mammogram revealed a shadow, leading to a breast cancer diagnosis that ultimately took her life. I still grieve for Carla, wishing I had known then what I know now. Perhaps she would still be with us.

Remember, every choice you make—from the food you eat to the products you use—is an opportunity to protect your hormonal health. In a world awash with xenoestrogens, your informed decisions are your best defense. Start making changes today and you'll be taking a vital step toward hormonal balance and well-being.

Magnesium: The Essential Mineral Powering over Three Hundred Bodily Functions

Magnesium is a cornerstone of optimal health, playing a vital role in many biological functions. It aids over 600 enzyme reactions in your body, so it's needed for many bodily processes. One of its main functions is to help produce ATP.

You can fix all the things that harm your mitochondria but without enough magnesium, your body can't make ATP from its precursor, adenosine diphosphate (ADP). This happens at complex V in the mitochondrial electron transport chain. Magnesium also helps maintain normal nerve and muscle function. It regulates neurotransmitters and makes sure nerves and muscles communicate well, which is vital for heartbeats and muscle relaxation, and overall cardiovascular health.

Additionally, magnesium plays a central role in bone health. It helps regulate calcium levels, ensuring calcium goes into the bones, not soft tissues, where it can cause harm. Magnesium's influence extends to blood sugar control as well. It enhances insulin sensitivity, helping to maintain stable blood glucose levels. This function is particularly important if you have or are at risk for diabetes.

Moreover, magnesium supports a healthy immune system. It helps control your immune response and keeps inflammation in check, boosting white blood cells that fight pathogens.

Unfortunately, it's hard to get enough magnesium from your diet. Soils have widespread nutrient deficiencies. Even if you consume plenty of leafy greens, the magnesium content may be suboptimal because much of our food is grown in depleted soils. This deficiency can lead to various health issues, such as muscle cramps, fatigue, and irregular heartbeats. To reduce the risk of deficiency, buy produce from biodynamic farms that regenerate their soil. Yet even taking actions such as these, many people still need magnesium supplements to meet their needs.

For adult men, the recommended dietary allowance (RDA) is 400–420 milligrams per day; for adult women, it is 310–320 milligrams per day. Pregnant women need about 350–360 milligrams per day. These amounts help ensure that your body's physiological needs are met.

When supplementing with magnesium, it's hard to go overboard. You don't need to be careful about every milligram. The ideal dose really depends on how much calcium you're taking in. For most folks, taking anywhere from 300 to 500 milligrams of magnesium a day can do wonders. But don't be afraid to go higher if you need to. A good rule of thumb is to aim for at least half the amount of your total calcium intake from all sources. If you're getting 1,000 milligrams of calcium, you might want to consider around 500 milligrams of magnesium.

Your body has a clever way of letting you know if you're taking too much magnesium—your stools will become loose. Don't worry, though; it's not dangerous. Just dial back your dose until things normalize again.

It's all about finding that sweet spot that works for your body. Everyone's different, so pay attention to how you feel and adjust accordingly. The goal is to give your body the magnesium it needs to thrive, without going overboard. It's a balancing act, but with a little attention, you'll find the right dose for you.

Niacinamide: Essential for Energy Production and Longevity

Niacinamide, also known as nicotinamide, is a form of niacin (vitamin B3) that plays a crucial role in energy metabolism. It is vital for your cells' energy production, keeping your mitochondrial electron transport chain working. Without enough niacinamide, your mitochondria can't make ATP.

The power of niacinamide lies in its ability to boost NAD+ (nicotinamide adenine dinucleotide). NAD+ helps convert food to energy; maintains DNA, gene expression, and redox balance; and also fuels sirtuins, which regulate longevity and metabolic health. NAD+ tends to deplete with age.

Niacinamide can also protect against PUFAs (polyunsaturated fatty acids) by inhibiting lipolysis, the breakdown of fats stored in fat cells. This anti-lipolytic effect prevents a rapid release of PUFAs into your bloodstream. In the blood, PUFAs can be oxidized, causing more oxidative stress and inflammation. Niacinamide helps manage the influx of harmful fats and slows the release of PUFAs from fat stores, which reduces the fats' availability for oxidation and damage.

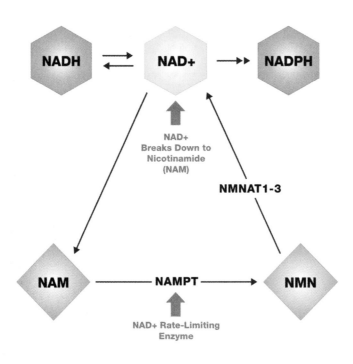

NAD+ metabolism cycle. When your body uses NAD+, it breaks down into niacinamide (NAM). The recycling process then begins. Niacinamide is converted to nicotinamide mononucleotide (NMN). NMN is then transformed back into NAD+. This is why niacinamide is such an effective NAD+ precursor.

The protective effects of niacinamide against chronic diseases are truly remarkable. Niacinamide can fight obesity and insulin resistance by reprogramming fat cells and boosting mitochondria. For neurodegeneration, it can boost energy in brain cells. It protects against damage and cognitive decline in Alzheimer's and Parkinson's diseases. In heart health, it helps maintain ATP production, which prevents stress from releasing profibrotic mediators that cause heart failure.

Niacinamide also helps with leaky gut syndrome, low testosterone, and kidney and liver diseases. It can reduce cortisol levels, thus reducing your stress. It aids in cancer prevention and treatment. It boosts your resilience against viruses, including COVID-19, and even helps treat glaucoma.

When it comes to dosing, I recommend that you use a low-dose daily regimen of 50 milligrams taken three times a day. This dose boosts your NAD+ levels far better than expensive newer options like NMN (nicotinamide mononucleotide) and NR (nicotinamide riboside). Niacinamide is incredibly cost-effective at only about twenty-five cents a month if you get it as a powder. Typically $1/64$ teaspoon of niacinamide powder is about 50 milligrams.

It's important to note the difference between niacinamide and niacin. While both are classified as vitamin B3, niacin doesn't activate the rate-limiting enzyme of NAD+ like niacinamide does. Also, niacinamide doesn't cause the flushing that niacin does. So, niacinamide provides more benefits with fewer side effects.

In my clinical practice, I've seen amazing results from niacinamide supplementation. One patient came to me struggling with chronic fatigue and early signs of cognitive decline. After starting her on a niacinamide regimen, we saw a boost in her energy and mental clarity within weeks. It's experiences like these that reinforce my belief in the power of this simple yet potent supplement.

NAD+ Testing: Unlocking the Secrets of Your Cellular Health
Testing your NAD+ level is a powerful tool in understanding your cellular health, but it's not as straightforward as you might think. NAD+ is very unstable when removed from your cells, which makes

it hard to measure accurately. This instability means samples must be handled with care and processed quickly to prevent degradation.

Typically, to get an accurate NAD+ measurement, you need to have your blood drawn in the same research laboratory where the testing occurs. This process often requires specialized equipment and techniques that aren't available in standard medical facilities. Transporting samples for NAD+ measurement risks damaging them, leading to very inaccurate results. The need for quick processing in a controlled environment makes it hard to measure this vital metabolic molecule.

But don't let these challenges discourage you. As a health pioneer, I've always believed in finding solutions where others see obstacles. That's why my team and I have developed a groundbreaking new test that sidesteps these difficulties. Measuring NAD+ directly is technically challenging, so we've created a method to measure your NAD+ levels indirectly. It assesses the redox state of three different molecules in your body.

Our test looks at the redox balance between acetoacetate and beta-hydroxybutyrate, lactate and pyruvate, and the oxidized and reduced forms of glutathione. These molecules are reliable indicators of your NAD+ status. They provide a powerful picture of your cellular health without the need for complex and costly direct NAD+ tests.

One of the most exciting aspects of this new test is its accessibility. We've worked hard to make it affordable, aiming to offer it at the same rate as our popular gut microbiome test. This means that more people can now check their NAD+ levels.

But why should you care about your NAD+ levels in the first place? Well, NAD+ is at the heart of nearly every aspect of your health. It's crucial for energy production, DNA repair, gene expression, and cellular stress response. As you age, your NAD+ levels decline. Many researchers believe that maintaining healthy NAD+ levels is key to healthy aging and longevity.

Testing your NAD+ levels gives you more than a number. It shows how well your cells are working—that is, how efficiently they're producing energy and repairing damage. This information is vital for anyone keen on optimizing their health and extending their healthy lifespan.

This test also allows you to verify the improvements you've made by following my recommendations. It's one thing to say these strategies will boost your mitochondria; it's another to show you the results in your body.

I've seen firsthand how powerful this kind of information can be. One of my patients was skeptical about the impact of my recommended lifestyle changes. But after seeing the dramatic improvement in his NAD+ levels after just a few months, he became a true believer. The data motivated him to stick with the program. You can find more information about this groundbreaking test at Mercola.com/tests. I encourage you to take advantage of this opportunity to gain deeper insights into your cellular health. Remember, knowledge is power when it comes to your health. Knowing your NAD+ status helps you make informed decisions.

In the world of health optimization, staying ahead of the curve is crucial. This NAD+ test represents the cutting edge of health assessment, offering you a window into the very core of your cellular function. Don't wait for problems to arise—take control of your health today by understanding and optimizing your NAD+ levels.

Thiamine's Role in Energy Metabolism and Neurological Function

Thiamine, or vitamin B1, is a vital nutrient for energy metabolism and nerve function. It's a water-soluble vitamin that your body doesn't store much of, which means you need to get it regularly from your diet or supplements. I've seen how treating thiamine deficiency can transform lives, so I'm excited to share this knowledge with you.

At its core, thiamine functions as a coenzyme in the form of thiamine pyrophosphate (TPP). This may sound like complex biochemistry, but it just means that TPP is essential for several enzymes in carbohydrate metabolism. Your cells use three enzymes to produce energy: pyruvate dehydrogenase, alpha-ketoglutarate dehydrogenase, and transketolase. These enzymes are the workhorses of the process.

Think of these enzymes as key players in an intricate relay race happening inside your cells. They're involved in the Krebs cycle and the pentose phosphate pathway, both critical for ATP production, the energy currency of your cells. Without adequate thiamine, the runners stumble and your energy production suffers.

One of the most crucial roles of thiamine is in glucose metabolism. Here's a key point that many people miss: your body doesn't burn glucose directly in the mitochondria. It must be broken down first, and this process requires thiamine. If you don't have enough thiamine, glucose won't properly burn in your mitochondria, leading to a buildup of pyruvate and lactate. This not only reduces ATP production but also contributes to cellular stress and dysfunction.

Thiamine is also essential for proper nerve cell function and neurotransmitter synthesis. Thiamine helps maintain the myelin sheath that insulates nerve fibers and lets nerves send impulses quickly. A lack of thiamine can break down this protective coating, leading to serious neurological problems.

One of the most well-known conditions that can benefit from thiamine supplementation is beriberi, which comes in two forms. Wet beriberi, which affects the heart and blood vessels, causes heart failure, edema, and shortness of breath. Dry beriberi, which impacts the nervous system, leads to neuropathy, muscle weakness, and even paralysis.

Another severe condition linked to thiamine deficiency is Wernicke-Korsakoff syndrome, often seen in those who suffer from chronic alcoholism. It has two paths: Wernicke's encephalopathy is a neurological disorder that causes confusion, ataxia, and eye movement issues, while Korsakoff's psychosis causes severe memory problems and confabulation. High-dose thiamine therapy can quickly relieve symptoms and even reverse neurological damage if caught early.

But it's not just these extreme conditions that benefit from thiamine. I've seen remarkable improvements in patients with type 2 diabetes when we address their thiamine status. Thiamine can boost glucose metabolism. It may lower the risk of complications from diabetes, such as neuropathy and heart disease. It shows promise in treating metabolic syndrome, a cluster of conditions that raise the risk of heart disease, stroke, and type 2 diabetes.

Heart failure patients can also benefit from thiamine supplementation. Studies have demonstrated that thiamine can improve heart function and reduce symptoms in these patients. This is likely due to its role in optimizing ATP production and supporting myocardial energy metabolism.

Emerging research suggests thiamine may also help brain function, reducing the risk of cognitive decline from aging and metabolic disorders, including Alzheimer's disease.

The recommended daily intake of thiamine varies depending on age, gender, and life stage. For infants, it starts at 0.2 milligrams for those aged 0–6 months and increases to 0.3 milligrams for those aged 7–12 months. As children grow, their thiamine needs increase: ages 1–3 need 0.5 milligrams daily; ages 4–8 need 0.6 milligrams; ages 9–13 need 0.9 milligrams per day.

For adolescents and adults, the recommendations further differ by gender. Males aged 14 years and older are advised to consume 1.2 milligrams of thiamine daily. Females aged 14–18 years should aim for 1.0 milligrams daily, while those 19 years and older need slightly more at 1.1 milligrams per day. For pregnant and breastfeeding women, who need more nutrients, a daily intake of 1.4 milligrams is recommended to support their health and the health of their babies.

These recommendations are a good start. But, in my experience, many people need higher doses. This is especially true for those with chronic health issues or a history of poor nutrition or alcohol use.

I remember a patient—let's call her Alicia—who came to me with chronic fatigue, brain fog, and numbness in her extremities. Her conventional doctors had run many tests but couldn't find the root cause. When we tested her thiamine levels, they were critically low. After a few weeks of high-dose thiamine, Alicia's energy and mental clarity improved. The numbness in her extremities began to subside. It was like watching a wilted plant come back to life after being watered.

Thiamine deficiency can cause severe health problems. Our diet of processed foods means many people lack thiamine. And some medicines and conditions can interfere with thiamine absorption or deplete it.

As you can see, thiamine is a powerhouse vitamin, vital for energy, heart health, and brain health. So don't underestimate the impact of this simple B vitamin.

Calcium: So Much More Than a Bone Builder

Let's talk about calcium, the quiet champion of your body's mineral team. Yes, calcium is important for strong bones, but it performs many additional roles. After all, calcium is the most abundant mineral in your body, and Mother Nature doesn't waste resources. When something is this plentiful, you can bet it's critically important.

Calcium is stored in your bones and teeth, giving them strength and structure. But that's just the beginning. It's crucial for nerve function, muscle contraction, and blood clotting. It also helps control blood pressure. In fact, low dietary calcium can increase your blood pressure by affecting the tone of your arteries.

Adequate calcium intake also reduces your risk of iron overload. This is significant because excess iron is associated with elevated levels of parathyroid hormone (PTH). PTH causes lactic acid production to help dissolve bone. It blocks the Krebs cycle, pushing your cells to glycolysis and suppressing carbon dioxide. This shift from producing carbon dioxide to lactate raises the pH in cells and increases the negative charge of cell proteins.

The result? Enhanced affinity for metals with a positive charge, such as iron, aluminum, and lead. These metals then accumulate in the soft tissues with calcium, causing calcification and forming lipofuscin, a sign of aging and a marker for senescent cells. The more calcium deficient you are, the more PTH is released, resulting in greater storage of these metals. It's a vicious cycle, but one you can break with proper calcium intake.

Calcium also plays defense for your body. It protects against lead toxicity by decreasing gastrointestinal lead absorption. Plus, it reduces oxalate absorption, which can be a problematic antinutrient if overconsumed. It's like calcium is your body's bouncer, keeping the troublemakers out.

Where can you get this wonder mineral? The best sources of calcium are not supplements but dairy products and cooked collard greens. Dairy products include milk, cottage cheese, Greek yogurt, and cheese. But here's a source you might not have considered: eggshells. Why? Eggshells are almost entirely composed of calcium carbonate and are an excellent natural source of calcium. They also contain twenty-seven other minerals that boost absorption. Plus, they have lower levels of toxic heavy metals than sources such as bone meal powder.

I know what you're thinking: "Dr. Mercola, are you seriously suggesting I eat eggshells?" Well, yes, I am. But don't worry—I'm not asking you to just crunch on some shells. There's a simple way to prepare them. Start by collecting clean eggshells. Rinse them thoroughly to remove any residual egg white or yolk, then place them in a pot of boiling water for about ten minutes to sterilize them.

After boiling, spread the eggshells on a baking sheet. Bake them at 200°F (93°C) for about fifteen minutes to dry them out. Once they're dry and brittle, transfer them to a coffee grinder and grind them into a fine powder. Make sure no sharp edges or large pieces remain. Store the eggshell powder in an airtight container, and add it to smoothies or sprinkle it on your food.

Having about a ½ teaspoon of powdered eggshell three times a day with meals will provide 1,300 milligrams of calcium. This is a great starting point if you're not consuming much raw dairy or cheese. If you experience constipation, supplement with magnesium at the same time. Most people will benefit from 2 to 4 grams of calcium a day combined from all these sources.

If you are concerned about the risk of calcification—the buildup of calcium in soft tissues and arteries—let me clear up a common misconception. It's low calcium intake, not high, that's the real culprit behind calcification. When you don't get enough calcium in your diet, your body goes into survival mode and starts pulling calcium from your bones, weakening them. At the same time, it raises calcium levels in your soft tissues. Over time, this can lead to those harmful deposits everyone's so worried about. It's a classic case of robbing Peter to pay Paul, and your body is stuck in the middle.

Are You Getting Too Much Phosphate? Here's Why It Matters for Your Health

There's another crucial aspect of calcium intake: its relationship with phosphate. Maintaining a balance between calcium and phosphate is important for optimal health. Phosphate, a charged particle containing phosphorus bound to oxygen, is abundant in meat, seeds, beans, nuts, whole grains, and processed foods. Modern diets have raised phosphate intake, but calcium intake has not risen as much.

This imbalance can trigger many health issues, including osteoporosis, high blood pressure, and calcification in the arteries and soft tissues. It may also cause metabolic disorders and central obesity. It can lead to hyperthyroidism, kidney stones, neurodegenerative diseases, and accelerated aging. The ideal calcium-to-phosphate ratio should be between 1:1 and 1.3:1. Phosphate is much more common in the Western diet than calcium, so it's even more important to get enough calcium.

My patient Richard was a corporate manager in Chicago. He loved his job, but his hectic lifestyle led to some unhealthy habits. He often relied on fast food and snacks to get through his busy days. He was unaware of the high phosphate levels in these foods. His favorite go-to items were colas, packaged meats, and microwaveable meals—all of which were loaded with hidden phosphates.

Over time, Richard noticed some troubling changes in his health. He felt constantly fatigued, his bones ached, and he suffered from frequent headaches. At first, he chalked it up to stress and getting older, but the symptoms persisted and worsened. A routine checkup showed high phosphate levels in his blood. His doctor said too much dietary phosphate could harm his health, weakening his bones, causing kidney problems, and raising his heart disease risk.

Alarmed by the diagnosis, Richard decided to change his diet and lifestyle because his calcium supplements were barely making a dent in his skewed calcium-to-phosphate ratio. We worked on reducing his phosphate intake while increasing his calcium from whole food sources. Six months later, his bone density had improved and he reported feeling more energetic and clearheaded.

Richard's case shows that it's about not just calcium intake but also balancing calcium with other nutrients, especially phosphate. It's not enough to just pop a calcium supplement and call it a day. You need to look at your diet and consider the interplay of various nutrients.

We can see that calcium is far more than just a bone builder and that a diet high in calcium from whole foods is key.

Eating dairy, leafy greens, and even eggshells will strengthen your bones and support your health. Check the quality of your calcium sources, especially cheese, and balance your calcium with phosphate.

Fine-Tuning Your Nutrient Orchestra

Your body is a complex system, and nutrients like the ones we covered in this chapter don't work in isolation. They're part of a grand orchestra, and when they're in balance, your health can play beautiful music.

To make sure you're not over- or underdoing it on any supplement we've covered, and that they are in proportion to each other, work with a health-care provider and check your levels every six months. And know that you are not just consuming supplements. You are taking an active role in your health—the key to long-term wellness and vitality.

CHAPTER 12

Empowering Your Metabolism: A Monthlong Journey to Vibrant Health

Now it's time to get started on implementing all the strategies I've covered in this book. To help you do that, I've outlined a four-week plan to optimize your metabolic health. This program focuses on a different lifestyle aspect each week that will help you unlock your body's full potential. By the end, you'll have a deeper understanding of your unique needs and form new habits that promote optimal metabolic function. I will provide you with a quick overview of the four-week plan and then we will dive deeper into the details. I suggest you keep this book handy for quick reference and spend some time on the same day each week to reread the plan for the week ahead. Also, before you begin the program, be sure to scan the QR code at end of chapter and download the free Mercola Health Coach app. This tool provides personalized guidance and evidence-based resources. It tracks your progress based on your health profile and uses nutritional science and lifestyle tips to boost your success in the program.

Getting on the Path to Better Health: The Four-Week Outline

- **Week 1: Laying the Foundation**

  Your first week is crucial. It focuses on preparation, assessing your diet, and clearing out unhealthy foods. I provide sample shopping lists and teach you how to assess your gut health and metabolic status. Calculating your daily caloric needs is an important task this week as undereating slows your metabolism and hurts your health goals. You'll also begin taking daily fifteen-minute walks, either in the early morning or late evening. High-intensity sun exposure should be avoided until or unless you've been seed oil–free for six months. You'll also add in small bursts of movement—what I call "exercise snacks"—throughout your day.

- **Week 2: Putting Plans Into Action**

  Now that your foundation is set, this week is about crafting balanced meals. They should have the right mix of fats, proteins, and carbs, with an emphasis on healthy carbs to efficiently fuel your cells. In week 2, you'll increase those daily walks to thirty minutes, continue your exercise snacks, and start prepping to add strength training in week 3.

- **Week 3: Strength in Motion**

  As you enter week three, you'll introduce strength training into your routine. This is essential for muscle building and improving cellular energy production, as muscle mass boosts your resting metabolic rate and insulin sensitivity. If you're new to strength training, start with bodyweight exercises or light weights, focusing on proper form and gradually increasing the difficulty level over time. You'll also extend your daily walks to forty-five minutes—still avoiding solar noon until you've been seed oil–free for six months—and keep up your exercise snacks. Follow the 80/20 rule to maintain balance in your routine: strive to make healthy choices 80 percent of the time, allowing for some flexibility in the remaining 20 percent. By week's end, you should feel more energetic, sleep better, and feel healthier. This indicates a more efficient metabolism.

- **Week 4: Reassessment Week**

  In this final week of the program, you'll reassess your gut health to see if food intolerances have decreased, digestion has improved, bloating is less frequent, and bowel movements are more regular. These indicators show your progress and areas for improvement. You'll also measure your metabolic rate again by taking many daily body temperature readings and comparing them to your initial baseline. Higher post-meal temperatures suggest improved metabolic efficiency. Then you'll gradually reintroduce eliminated foods one at a time, monitoring for any digestive issues or energy changes. Keep a food diary to track the reintroductions and their effects.

  During this week you'll also bump up your daily walk to one hour and add an additional strength-training session.

Now let's take a closer look at what happens in each of these four weeks.

Week 1: Prepping for Change

Although the focus for week 1 is on food, there are a few other things you can do to set yourself up for success. Let's start with movement. Begin each day with a fifteen-minute walk in the morning before 10:00 a.m. or after 4:00 p.m. You will need to be off all vegetable oils for four to six months before it is safe for you to sunbathe around solar noon.

The simple habit of a daily walk serves many purposes. It gets your body moving, helps regulate your circadian rhythm, and lets you soak up some natural vitamin D. These are crucial for your metabolic health.

In addition to these brief walks, look for opportunities to incorporate "exercise snacks" throughout your day. These brief bursts of physical activity include taking the stairs instead of the elevator, doing a few squats while waiting for your coffee to brew, or stretching during commercial breaks when watching TV. The goal is to keep your body moving and grooving all day long.

Next, let's focus on optimizing your sleep environment. Quality sleep is key to metabolic health. A major disruptor of sleep today is excessive blue light, especially at night. To combat this, consider swapping out your regular light bulbs for red ones in the areas where you spend your evenings. Or invest in a pair of blue-blocking glasses to wear in the hours leading up to bedtime.

Don't forget about your electronic devices. On your phone, tablet, and computer, install apps or adjust settings to reduce blue-light emission in the evenings. These small changes can have a significant impact on your sleep quality and, by extension, your metabolic health.

Foods to Eliminate

As you seek to boost your cellular energy, what you don't eat is just as important as what you do eat. Certain foods can harm your mitochondria, so you'll want to avoid them to support your metabolic health.

First on the chopping block are seed oils and vegetable oils, such as sunflower oil, canola oil, soy oil, corn oil, sesame oil, and grapeseed oil. These oils are high in polyunsaturated fats (PUFAs) that disrupt your body's ability to burn carbs efficiently. Instead, opt for more stable cooking fats like butter, ghee, or coconut oil.

Next, it's time to bid farewell to dairy alternatives like almond milk and oat milk. These products often contain additives and lack the nutritional benefits of real dairy. If you tolerate dairy well, choose organic, ideally raw milk from grass-fed cows. If not, focus on other nutrient-dense foods to meet your nutritional needs.

You should also eliminate all flax products—including flax seeds, flax oil, and flax-based foods. While often touted as a health food, flax can interfere with hormone balance due to its high phytoestrogen content. The same goes for soy products—avoid tofu, edamame, soy milk, and soy protein powder.

Veggie burgers seem healthy, but many store-bought options are full of processed ingredients and unhealthy oils. If you eat meat, choose high-quality, grass-fed beef or bison. If you're vegetarian or vegan, eat whole food, plant-based proteins that are balanced. You frequently need to combine proteins from different sources to obtain a complete set of amino acids.

Whey protein powder is another item to remove from your diet. While it's a popular supplement, it can be hard on your digestion and lacks the balanced amino acid profile found in whole-food protein sources. Replace it with bone broth or collagen powder for a more easily digestible and beneficial protein source.

Lastly, cut all products containing high-fructose corn syrup. This highly processed sweetener has been linked to health issues and has no nutritional value. If you need to sweeten foods, opt for small amounts of maple syrup, raw honey, or organic cane sugar instead. Do not use artificial sweeteners as they're all toxic to one degree or another.

Foods to Limit

While you need to eliminate some foods entirely, others can be consumed in moderation. These foods aren't harmful in small amounts, but overconsumption can hurt your metabolic health goals.

Olive oil, often considered a healthy fat, is high in monounsaturated fats (MUFAs). Excessive MUFA intake sends hibernation signals to your body that downregulate your metabolism, making it harder to lose weight. Despite being better than PUFAs, use it sparingly, if at all.

Nuts, seeds, and their butters fall into a similar category. While they contain beneficial nutrients, they're also high in PUFAs and can be easy to overeat. If you include them, do so only in small amounts and not daily.

Chia seeds, despite their popularity as a superfood, are also high in PUFAs. Include them occasionally but don't make them a staple in your diet.

Hummus and chickpeas, while not necessarily harmful, are also best limited due to their PUFA content. If you enjoy them, consume them in moderation, but do not eat them every day.

When it comes to animal products, be mindful of the source. Confinement-raised chicken, eggs, and pork often come from animals fed high-PUFA diets, which affects the meat's nutritional composition. Choose pasture-raised options whenever possible, and if you only have access to conventionally raised animal products, make them an occasional part of your diet and not a daily staple.

Cold-water fatty fish and fish oils, while rich in omega-3s, are also high in PUFAs. Include them in your diet occasionally, but do not rely on them as your primary protein source.

Avocados and avocado oil, like olive oil, are high in MUFAs. They have some health benefits but eat them in moderation. Too much can signal your body to enter hibernation mode.

Some protein sources, such as chicken breasts and beef tenderloin, are high in amino acids like tryptophan and methionine, which can suppress your metabolism. It's best to limit these cuts of meat and focus more on collagen-rich protein sources.

Store-bought baked goods and bread often contain unhealthy oils. They are also made with iron-fortified flour, which can harm gut health. If you include bread in your diet, opt for homemade sourdough or other minimally processed options.

Finally, raw vegetables can be tough on weak digestive systems due to their high fiber content. If you have gut issues, it's best to thoroughly cook most of your vegetables until your digestion improves.

Assess Your Gut Health

Your gut health plays a crucial role in your well-being and metabolic function. To get a clear picture of your current gut health, it is important to assess your digestive symptoms. Start by answering these four questions:

1. Do you have a long list of food intolerances? If you can only tolerate a very limited set of foods, this could be a sign of compromised gut health.

2. Do you experience bloating or stomach pain after eating foods that contain fiber, such as fruits, potatoes, or vegetables? This might indicate an inability to process certain types of carbohydrates.

3. Do you have a bowel movement every day? Ideally you should have at least one per day. If you find yourself going every other day or less frequently, this could be a sign of digestive issues.

4. Do you suffer from chronic diarrhea? Persistent loose stools can be a sign of inflammation or other gut problems.

If you answered yes to at least three of these four questions, your gut is likely in a highly compromised state. Don't worry, though—this doesn't mean you're doomed. Your gut has an incredible ability to heal, and with the right approach, you'll be on your way to better digestive health.

In cases of severely compromised gut health, you might need what I call a "Metabolic Boost." This is a targeted approach to jump-start your gut healing process, which we'll cover in week 2 of the program. The Metabolic Boost includes specific diets and supplements aimed at recovering your gut health and optimizing your metabolism.

Remember, everyone's gut-health journey is unique. The goal is to gradually become less restrictive with your diet as your gut health improves. By assessing your current state, you're taking the first step toward a healthier, more resilient digestive system.

Assess Your Metabolic Rate

Now that you've evaluated your gut health, it's time to assess your metabolic rate. Your body temperature is a good indicator of how well your body creates and uses energy. Higher body temperatures usually mean a higher metabolic rate. Energy production generates heat.

To assess your metabolic health, measure your body temperature several times a day. Use an inexpensive oral thermometer under your tongue. Avoid using ear or forehead thermometers as they're less accurate for this purpose.

Here's when to measure your body temperature:

1. Immediately upon waking

2. Forty minutes after breakfast

3. Forty minutes after lunch

In a healthy body, your waking temperature should be in the high 97°F to low 98°F range. After each meal, your temperature should gradually rise, reaching 98.6°F by midday or early afternoon, and then slowly decline as you get closer to bedtime.

Ideally your temperature should rise after breakfast, indicating effective energy production from food. If your temperature falls after breakfast, it could be due to elevated stress hormones such as cortisol and adrenaline, in the morning. It might also indicate an underactive thyroid.

To make it easier to keep track of your body temperature, use the Mercola Health Coach app. This handy tool allows you to record your temperature readings easily and helps you understand your metabolic trends. The app will track your measurements over time so you can see how your metabolic rate changes as you implement the strategies detailed in this program.

Don't be discouraged if your initial readings show a low metabolic rate. Your body can heal itself. The diet and lifestyle changes in this program can boost your metabolism. As you become more efficient at converting food into energy (ATP), your body temperature will rise.

Assess Your Daily Caloric Needs

Meeting your daily caloric needs—without overindulging—is crucial for optimizing your metabolic health. Chronic undereating can signal starvation to your body, which will slow your metabolism to save energy. This is counterproductive when your goal is to maximize cellular energy production and heal your body.

To estimate your calorie needs, multiply your ideal weight in pounds by 11 if you are a man and 10 if you are a woman (for kilograms, use 24 for men and 21.6 for women). Fine-tune this by multiplying by 1.2 if you are sedentary, 1.3 if you are active, and 1.5 if you are very active.

Remember to use your ideal weight, not your current weight, for this calculation. This ensures that you're providing your body with the right amount of fuel for optimal function without excess calories.

Avoid very low-calorie diets as they can be detrimental to your metabolic health. Your body will not thrive if you're consistently eating less than 1,800 calories per day. As your metabolism improves, you'll burn more calories. As your body becomes better at turning food into energy, you'll be able to eat more without gaining weight.

If you've been on a very-low-calorie diet, don't jump to a drastic increase. Instead, slowly ramp up your intake by about 50 calories per day each week. Monitor your weight trends (not daily fluctuations) to ensure you're not moving too quickly. The goal is to find your maintenance calorie range, which is the highest number of calories you can consume without gaining weight.

If you're switching from a low-carb or keto diet, you might gain weight when reintroducing carbs. This is normal and primarily due to increased water retention as your body replenishes its glycogen stores. Don't be alarmed by this initial fluctuation—focus on how you feel and your health markers.

To track your food intake and meet your calorie and nutrient needs, I recommend the Food Buddy app, which is part of the Mercola Health Coach app. This tool allows you to log your meals, track your macronutrient ratios, and monitor your progress over time.

Simply take a picture of the QR code at the end of this chapter with your cell phone to get free access to this valuable app.

Make a Shopping List

Now that you've checked your gut health and metabolic rate, it's time to stock your kitchen with the right foods for your metabolic recovery. Creating a well-thought-out shopping list is key to setting yourself up for success. Remember, when you fail to plan, you plan to fail.

Your shopping list should include a variety of nutrient-dense foods across different categories. Here's a breakdown of what to include:

Carbs and Fresh Produce

- Seasonal, ripe fruits
- A variety of vegetables (choose based on your current gut health)
- Herbs and spices for flavoring
- Raw honey, maple syrup, or organic cane sugar (use sparingly)
- Organic potatoes and/or sweet potatoes
- Organic sourdough bread or organic wheat and/or rye flour for making your own sourdough
- Organic white rice

Fats

- Butter (preferably from grass-fed cows)
- Tallow or ghee for cooking

- Coconut oil
- Eggs from pasture-raised chickens
- Raw cheese (ideally made with animal rennet)

Proteins

- Ground beef or bison (grass-fed, if possible)
- Gelatinous cuts of meat, such as beef shank, oxtail, or skirt steak
- Collagen or gelatin powder
- Raw milk (if tolerated and available in your area)
- Knuckle bones or "soup bones" for making bone broth

When choosing produce, look for organic options. For animal products, opt for pasture-raised and grass-fed options when available and within your budget.

Remember, you don't need to buy everything on this list. Choose a mix of nutrient-dense foods that align with your gut health and dietary preferences. The goal is to have a well-stocked kitchen that supports your new healthy eating habits.

As you shop, be mindful of reading labels and avoiding foods with added sugars, unhealthy oils, or artificial ingredients. Stick to the perimeter of the grocery store where fresh, whole foods are typically found.

With your shopping list and your kitchen stocked with metabolic-friendly foods, you're ready to start your journey to better health. Remember, small, consistent changes add up to significant improvements over time. Be patient with yourself and celebrate each step you take toward a healthier, more vibrant you.

Get More Movement

This week you want to begin taking a fifteen-minute walk every day, taking care to avoid going outside at solar noon until you have been off seed oils for six months. Taking your walk in the morning not only helps regulate your circadian rhythm but also boosts your vitamin D levels and energy. If the dangers of seed oils were already on your radar before reading this book, and you've already curtailed your intake for a few months before starting this program, then great! Taking your daily walk at solar noon will provide you will all the benefits the sun has to offer with a reduced risk of skin damage. In addition to your daily walks, incorporate unlimited exercise snacks throughout your day: short walks, squats, lunges as you move between rooms, or push-ups during commercials.

The beauty of exercise snacks lies in their ability to stimulate your mitochondria, the powerhouses of your cells. By engaging in brief, intense bouts of activity, you're telling your body to ramp up energy production. This improves cellular efficiency, enhancing your overall metabolic health. You'll likely find that these short bursts of movement leave you feeling energized and focused rather than drained.

Week 1 Checklist

At the end of your first week of metabolic recovery, be sure to review your progress. Remember, this week was all about building a solid foundation for the weeks ahead. Let's go through a comprehensive checklist to make sure you're on track.

❑ Have you cleared out your kitchen of unhealthy food choices? This step is vital in setting yourself up for success. Remove any items that don't fit your new health goals, focusing on those high in unhealthy fats, added sugars, or processed ingredients.

❑ Have you established the habit of taking a daily fifteen-minute walk at midday—or at less sunny times if you're still eliminating seed oils? If you've missed a day or two, don't worry—just commit to making it a consistent part of your routine moving forward.

❑ Have you taken short movement breaks throughout the day?

❑ Have you invested in red light bulbs or blue-light-blocking glasses? If you haven't made this purchase yet, prioritize it for the coming week.

❑ Have you taken the time to honestly consider your digestive symptoms? This information will guide your dietary choices in the weeks to come, so be thorough and truthful in your assessment.

❏ Have you measured your body temperature to assess your metabolic health? Remember, this should be done at specific times throughout the day to get an accurate picture of your metabolic function.

❏ Have you calculated your daily caloric needs based on your ideal body weight? This number will serve as a guide as you adjust your diet in the coming weeks.

❏ Have you created a comprehensive shopping list and stocked up on the recommended foods? Having the right ingredients on hand will make it much easier to stick to your new eating plan.

Week 2: Implementation

As you move into week 2, it's time to put your plans into action. This week is all about implementation and building on the foundation you've created.

While strength training isn't on the agenda until week 3, now is the time to start planning for its introduction. Don't worry if you're new to strength training. Developing your personal routine doesn't have to be daunting or expensive. Start by reflecting on the types of exercises that appeal to you. Do you prefer bodyweight exercises you can do at home or are you drawn to using weights at a gym? Perhaps resistance bands or kettlebells intrigue you? Research different work-out routines and decide which approach resonates with you to ensure you're ready to hit the ground running next week.

Start your blue-light reduction strategies this week, like using those red light bulbs or blue-light-blocking glasses in the evening hours. Create a soothing bedtime routine that signals to your body that it's time to wind down. This might include dimming lights, avoiding electronic screens, or doing something relaxing, such as reading or gentle stretching.

Now is also the time to put your meal plans into practice. Start preparing and eating the balanced meals you've planned. (We'll cover how to create the right mix of proteins, fats, and carbs below.) Pay close attention to how different foods make you feel. Are you experiencing more energy? Better digestion? Make notes of these observations to guide future adjustments.

As you begin these dietary changes, keep embracing the 80/20 rule. Strive to make healthy choices 80 percent of the time. This approach helps support sustainability and prevents feelings of deprivation. Remember, progress is more important than perfection. If you have a less-than-ideal meal or day, don't get discouraged. Simply refocus and get back on track with your next meal.

Recommended Macronutrient Ratios

The right macronutrient balance is key to optimizing your metabolic health. Let's break down the recommended ratios:

- Protein should make up about 15 percent of your daily calories, calculated at 0.6–0.8 grams per pound of your ideal body weight. For example, if your ideal weight is 150 pounds, aim for 90–120 grams of protein daily. Remember, one-third of this protein should come from collagen-rich sources to support skin, joint, and gut health.

- Fat should make up 30–40 percent of your daily calories. This might seem lower than some popular high-fat diets, but your focus is on metabolic efficiency. Too much dietary fat can interfere with your body's ability to properly metabolize carbohydrates.

- Carbohydrates should make up the remaining 45–55 percent of your calories. This higher-carb approach may be new to you, but it's vital for fueling your cells and optimizing metabolic function.

Best Types of Protein

Not all protein sources are created equal when it comes to supporting metabolic health. Here are some top choices to include in your diet:

- Bone broth, collagen powder, and gelatin powder are excellent sources of collagen proteins. They support gut health, joint function, and skin elasticity.

- Ground beef and bison are nutrient-dense options, rich in minerals such as zinc and iron. They also contain a mix of muscle meat and connective tissue, providing a good balance of amino acids.

- Gelatinous cuts of meat such as beef shank, oxtail, and chicken gizzards are fantastic sources of collagen protein. These cuts need slow cooking to break down tough tissues, making for tender and tasty meals.

- Organic, grass-fed raw dairy has a complete protein profile. It also has beneficial fats and vitamins. If raw dairy isn't available or suitable for you, opt for minimally processed organic dairy.

- Organic, pasture-raised eggs are a superfood. They provide high-quality protein, vitamins, and minerals. Limit to three to four per day unless they are low-LA eggs.

- Organic, pasture-raised pork is high in protein and a top source of thiamine (vitamin B1), vital for energy metabolism.

- Low-fat, wild-caught seafood such as shrimp, scallops, cod, and mussels offer a unique amino acid profile and are rich in minerals from the sea.

Best Types of Fats

Choosing the right fats is crucial for refining your metabolic health. For cooking over high heat, opt for ghee and tallow. These saturated fats are stable at high temperatures, making them less likely to oxidize and form harmful compounds. For lower-temperature cooking or sautéing, butter and coconut oil are excellent choices.

When it comes to dietary fats, prioritize sources that are low in linoleic acid and have a higher ratio of saturated to monounsaturated fats. Top choices include:

- Butter or ghee: rich in beneficial fatty acids and fat-soluble vitamins

- Egg yolks: packed with nutrients and healthy fats

- Dairy fats from cheese, yogurt, and milk: they provide a good balance of saturated and monounsaturated fats

- Dark chocolate (without soy lecithin, high-fructose corn syrup, or artificial flavors): a tasty source of healthy fats and antioxidants

- Coconut oil: rich in medium-chain triglycerides (MCTs) that can boost metabolism

Remember, while these fats are healthy, moderation is key. Aim to keep your total fat intake within the recommended 30–40 percent of daily calories.

Best Types of Carbs

To optimize your metabolic health, you must know how carbs are categorized. There are two main types of carbs: simple and complex.

Simple carbs have one of two basic chemical structures:

- Monosaccharides (single sugar molecules), such as glucose and fructose

- Disaccharides (two sugar molecules linked together), such as sucrose in sugar and fruit, and lactose in milk

These simple carbs are easily digested by your body due to their uncomplicated structure. You'll find them in foods such as ripe fruit, fruit juice, honey, sugar, and maple syrup.

Complex carbs are made up of longer, more intricate chains of sugar molecules. These include oligosaccharides and polysaccharides. There are many different kinds of complex carbs, including:

1. **Fiber.** This is a type of complex carbohydrate that the human body cannot digest. Unlike starch, which is composed entirely of glucose molecules, dietary fibers can include a variety of other sugar molecules such as fructose, galactose, and mannose, depending on the type. Fibers are found in fruits, vegetables, grains, and legumes.

2. **Inulin.** A type of soluble fiber found in various plants, inulin is composed of fructose molecules instead of glucose. It is found in foods such as artichokes, garlic, onions, and asparagus. Inulin is often used as a prebiotic to stimulate the growth of beneficial bacteria in the gut.

3. **Pectins.** These are complex carbohydrates that are rich in galacturonic acid and found in the cell walls of plants, especially fruits. Pectins are used in food as gelling agents, particularly in jams and jellies.

4. **Beta-glucans**. Found in cereal grains like oats and barley, beta-glucans consist of glucose molecules linked in a specific way that is different from starch. They are known for their health benefits, including lowering cholesterol levels and improving heart health.

5. **Gums**. These are polysaccharides used in the food industry as thickening, stabilizing, or emulsifying agents. Examples include guar gum and xanthan gum, which are composed of sugars such as mannose and glucuronic acid.

6. **Starch**. A polysaccharide made up of glucose molecules that excels at replenishing muscle glycogen, starch is vital for muscle growth and recovery.

All complex carbs take longer to digest. This slower digestion process provides a more sustained release of energy compared to simple carbs.

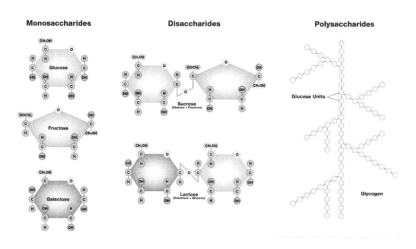

Structural representations of carbohydrates: monosaccharides, disaccharides, and polysaccharides.

The key to a balanced, metabolically supportive diet is to include both simple and complex sugars and starches. This approach makes your meals varied and enjoyable, and helps you stick to your new eating habits. It also gives you essential vitamins, minerals, and fiber. Each type of carbohydrate plays a unique and important role in your body's functioning.

For instance, fructose and glucose replenish liver glycogen faster than starches. This is beneficial for estrogen detoxification and the conversion of T4 into the active thyroid hormone T3, both of which occur in your liver. Starches, however, replenish muscle glycogen quickly, which helps your muscles grow and recover. They also send signals of abundance and homeostasis to your body, supporting metabolic health, so it's important to eat both types regularly.

To find the best carbs for your diet, test options from both columns in Table 1 below. Begin with the green-labeled items, which are generally well tolerated. Test the yellow-labeled items one by one. Carefully proceed with testing red-labeled options as it will likely take you some time to tolerate these carbs.

This system will help you find the best carbs to suit your digestion and microbiome. You can see how different carbs affect your body and then optimize your diet for your gut's current state.

Your gut health affects how well you tolerate different carbs, and your metabolic rate influences your gut health. As your cells produce more energy, you'll likely tolerate more foods. This is a clear sign of improving health.

CARBOHYDRATE SOURCES

Green	Yellow	Red
Dextrose	Maple Syrup	Non-Starchy Veggies
	Fruit Juice with Pulp	
White Rice	Whole Fruits	Starchy Veggies
	Custom Pasta	Beans and Legumes
Sucrose	Pulp-Free Fruit Juice	
	Root Veggies	Whole Grains

Classification of carbohydrate sources. This color-coded chart illustrates a strategic progression of carbohydrate sources, designed to support the rehabilitation of gut health and optimize energy production. The categorization is based on the complexity and digestibility of the carbohydrates.

Why Veggies Alone Aren't Enough

You might be wondering, "What about vegetables? Aren't they the cornerstone of a healthy diet?" Well-cooked vegetables should be part of a balanced diet, but they have limits in meeting your energy needs.

Vegetables are great sources of fiber, polyphenols, minerals, and vitamins such as vitamin K1. However, they're not high-energy or high-carb sources, which means you can't rely on vegetables alone to meet your body's energy requirements. No matter how many veggies you eat, they won't provide enough calories or carbohydrates to fuel optimal metabolic function.

Moreover, a diet that's excessively high in fiber but low in energy can lead to gut problems. If your gut lacks energy, it can't move fiber well. This can cause fermentation, gas, and harmful bacteria to grow. This, in turn, drives endotoxin production, potentially causing more harm than good.

So, while vegetables are important, it's crucial not to overdo it. Include vegetables you enjoy and tolerate. They provide vitamins, minerals, and fiber. But ensure a balanced diet with enough simple and complex carbs from other sources.

It's also worth noting that raw vegetables can be particularly challenging for your digestive system. Cooking vegetables not only makes them easier to digest but also enhances the availability of certain nutrients. Some great options to include in your diet are collard greens, beets, zucchini, squash, tomatoes, green beans, and turnips. Just remember to cook them well to ensure digestibility and nutrient absorption.

As you experiment with these meal ideas and create your own combinations, pay attention to how your body responds. Use your body temperature as a gauge for your metabolism. A rise in body temperature after meals means your metabolism is improving. Your body is upregulating nonessential tasks due to more energy.

Remember, aim for a waking body temperature in the high 97°F to low 98°F range. At midday, it should be 98.6°F, as a meal that boosts your metabolism should raise both heat and energy. A rise in body temperature signals improved energy production in your cells. And this boost in energy often reduces symptoms. As you continue this journey, you'll likely find that you're not just eating better but feeling better, too. Your energy levels may improve, your digestion may become more comfortable, and you may even find yourself enjoying food in a whole new way. This is the power of eating for metabolic health. It's not about restriction but about giving your body exactly what it needs to function at its best.

Meal-Planning Tips and Pointers

As you embark on your journey to optimal metabolic health, meal planning becomes a crucial tool in your arsenal. The goal is to regularly consume starch, which will help maximize your metabolic rate. When your metabolism is functioning well, you'll be able to eat a wide variety of foods without digestive issues—a clear sign of good health.

Start by identifying the fiber sources that work best for you. This is important for both gut health and adequate carb consumption. Not every food will agree with everyone, so listen to your body. Pay attention to how different carb sources, both simple sugars and starches, affect your digestion and energy levels. Your taste preferences and the availability of foods in your area will also play a role in deciding your ideal carb sources.

Timing Your Meals Properly Allows You to Sleep Better

- Limit meal frequency: Aim for three main meals a day instead of constant snacking.

- Restrict your eating window: confine eating to a twelve-hour period but not less than eight hours daily.

- Schedule your meals wisely: begin eating shortly after you wake in the morning; finish your last meal at least three hours before bedtime to support better sleep.

This approach helps your migrating motor complex (MMC), a series of muscle contractions in your gut that occurs between meals. The MMC helps prevent bacterial overgrowth by "cleaning up" your digestive tract when you're not eating. It's activated every two to three hours during fasting periods, so try to space your meals and snacks at least three hours apart.

Cook your meals at home most of the time. It's hard to eat out and support your metabolism when you have no control over the ingredients and how they are prepared. Cooking at home lets you use the best ingredients and methods to support metabolic health.

Remember, enjoying your food is crucial. I like to call this vitamin J for "Joy." It's an essential part of health and makes eating for cellular energy production sustainable in the long run. When you enjoy your meals, you're more likely to stick with your new eating habits.

It's fine to have weight-loss goals. But it's even better to focus on improving energy production. Eating enough calories and not gaining weight will boost your metabolism. This approach often leads to natural weight loss as your body becomes more efficient at using energy.

Tracking your food intake for a period can be incredibly insightful. It ensures you're eating enough and consuming appropriate amounts of each macronutrient. Many people, when not tracking their intake, tend to eat too much fat and too few carbs. This can hinder metabolic improvement.

Lastly, make sure you're including enough high-calcium sources, such as dairy products or well-cooked collard greens, in your diet. If needed, consider supplementing with eggshell powder. This will help ensure a balanced calcium-to-phosphorus ratio, which is vital for health and strong bones.

Sample Meal Plan

Now that you know to include various carbs in your diet, let's apply this to a sample meal plan. This plan is designed to provide inspiration and is by no means exhaustive. Each meal in this plan has a starch, a sucrose source, a healthy fat, collagen, and an animal protein. This combination helps ensure you're getting a good balance of nutrients to support your metabolic health.

- For breakfast, you might enjoy potatoes with cheese, eggs, and fruit. Have coffee with a bit of maple syrup or honey and a splash of milk or cream. Another option could be sourdough bread with marmalade, eggs, and bone broth, again with coffee sweetened naturally. For a savory breakfast, try breakfast tacos:

fill nixtamalized corn tortillas (or cassava tortillas or sourdough flour tortillas) with eggs and a cooked vegetable of your choice.

- Lunchtime offers plenty of delicious possibilities. One unique option is a Japanese sweet potato topped with dark chocolate, served alongside cheese and bone broth. This might sound unusual, but it's a favorite of Ashley Armstrong, the clinical consultant for this book. Alternatively, you could enjoy a bowl of white rice cooked in bone broth, topped with egg yolks and grated cheese, served with fruit or fruit juice. For a heartier lunch, try a braised beef shank stew with broth, potatoes, and your choice of vegetables, accompanied by fruit or fruit juice.

- For dinner, consider a meal of ground beef, bone broth, white rice with some butter or ghee, and well-cooked vegetables of your choice. Another option is a braised pork hock stew with collard greens, served with homemade cornbread made using masa harina. For a quick and easy dinner, try a "fried rice" dish using rice, butter or ghee, eggs, and your preferred vegetables, served with bone broth and fruit.

- Don't forget about snacks! Some ideas are cottage cheese with fruit and homemade gummies (made from fruit juice and gelatin powder), a simple mix of cheese and fruit, or milk with a bit of maple syrup for sweetness.

Week 2 Variation: The Metabolic Boost

For those with damaged guts who struggle to tolerate many foods, we have a special approach called the Metabolic Boost. This is a short-term plan to boost your metabolism and reactivate functions that may have slowed due to poor gut health.

The primary goal of the Metabolic Boost is to minimize gut disturbances while improving energy production. We do this by giving your body easy-to-digest carbs that support T4-to-T3 conversion and boost gut motility. You will limit fibers that irritate your digestive tract and gradually reintroduce more foods over time.

During the Metabolic Boost phase, you can use any of the recommended healthy fat and protein sources listed earlier. However, keep your fat intake moderate to low, as a high-fat approach can worsen endotoxin transport out of the gut. Prioritize collagen sources for your protein intake.

For carbohydrates, you'll need to gauge your own tolerance. You may find that simpler sugars are better tolerated than starches or certain fibers. That means prioritizing the green carb sources listed in chapter 10 (see page 253), minimizing the yellow and avoiding the red. Some of the best carbs to try include dextrose water, raw honey, maple syrup, organic sugar, ripe fruits, fruit juices, and well-cooked white rice. Boiled white button mushrooms with a dash of coconut oil, vinegar, and salt can help clear out debris in the intestines. The fiber in boiled mushrooms is usually well tolerated and won't cause disruption.

How Do You Know If You Need the Metabolic Boost? Look for These Signs

- Extreme food intolerances or a very limited set of tolerated foods
- Bloating or stomach pain after ingesting fiber sources
- Slow motility, chronic constipation, chronic diarrhea, or irregular bowel movements

A Sample Food Plan for the Metabolic Boost Phase

- Breakfast: 2–3 cups well-cooked organic white rice (brown rice has fiber that most do not tolerate well) with 1 scoop of collagen, 3 eggs, and coffee with 1–2 tablespoons organic sugar, maple syrup, or honey.
- Lunch: 2–3 cups well-cooked organic white rice, 1 cup well-cooked squash, 1 cup bone broth, and 4 ounces lightly cooked ground beef. Also, coffee with 1–2 tablespoons of organic sugar, maple syrup, or honey.
- Dinner: 1 cup boiled white button mushrooms with 1 teaspoon coconut oil, a dash of vinegar, and salt; 1 cup well-cooked white rice; 1 cup ripe fruit (if tolerated without causing gas or other GI issues); 1 cup bone broth; 1 serving aged A2 cheese.

- Snack: Homemade gummies made with 1 cup fruit juice and 10 grams gelatin powder.

During this phase, it's crucial to ensure a daily bowel movement. If needed, take ⅛–¼ teaspoon cascara sagrada at night before bed. Avoid hunger by adding more dextrose water or your preferred sugar source as necessary. If using sugar (dextrose) water, remember to sip it slowly over time.

To know when to end this phase, track your waking body temperature. You should see it rise over time, indicating improved metabolism. You'll also have more energy, regular bowel movements, and better food tolerance. As you improve, slowly add other carb sources.

Week 2 Checklist

As you wrap up week 2 of your health journey, use this checklist to ensure you've completed all the necessary steps:

- ❏ Are you taking a daily thirty-minute walk (up from the fifteen-minute walk in week 1)? And are you continuing to weave exercise snacks into your daily routine?

- ❏ Have you made a plan to add strength training next week?

- ❏ Are you reducing blue-light exposure at night?

- ❏ Have you created a balanced meal plan that meets your calorie needs and includes the best types of carbs, fats, and proteins in the appropriate ratios?

- ❏ Have you assessed your gut status to see if you should start with the Metabolic Boost phase?

- ❏ Are you following the 80/20 rule and remembering that it doesn't have to be perfect?

As always, keep in mind that this is a process and every small step counts. Be patient with yourself, celebrate your progress, and look forward to the positive changes ahead in week 3.

Week 3: Up the Ante

It's time to take your progress to the next level. You've laid the foundation for better health and now you're ready for more. In week

3 you'll push your boundaries and challenge yourself to achieve even greater results.

Extend Your Midday Walks

Your first task is to increase your daily walks to forty-five minutes. This simple yet powerful change will yield significant benefits. But remember, while the sunlight present at solar noon improves your health, it is smart to avoid it until your diet has been free of seed oils for six months. So, walk in the early morning or late afternoon or evening until you clear the seed oils from your skin.

As you go on these longer walks, take time to appreciate the world around you. Notice the subtle changes in your environment: the rustle of leaves, the warmth of sunlight on your skin, the rhythm of your breath. Simultaneously tune in to your body and observe the positive changes happening within. You might feel increased energy, improved mental clarity, or a general sense of well-being.

Add Morning Sunlight Exposure

You've improved your evening routine to cut blue light before bed. Now let's optimize your mornings. As soon as you wake up, aim to get some sunlight exposure. If this happens on your daily walk, that is great, but if you don't have time for a forty-five-minute walk in the morning, aim for at least ten minutes of sun exposure. This simple habit can greatly improve your circadian rhythm, boosting your sleep quality and health.

Start by standing outside and looking in the direction of the sun for just one minute. As you become more comfortable with this routine, try to extend it to ten minutes. This morning light exposure sends a powerful signal to your body, indicating that it's time to be alert and active. It helps regulate your cortisol levels, improving your energy and focus throughout the day.

Weave in Strength Training

The most exciting addition to week 3 is the introduction of strength training. Dedicate thirty minutes once a week to resistance exercises.

Once you've identified your preferred exercise types, if you're not training with a professional in the gym, use YouTube as your personal trainer. Explore different channels and instructors. Watch a variety of videos on the exercises you're interested in. Pay close attention to the instructors' cues about proper form, breathing techniques, and common mistakes to avoid. Remember, the goal isn't to become an expert overnight. Start small. Master a few basic exercises. Then, expand your repertoire as you gain confidence and strength.

Week 3 Checklist

As you wrap up week 3, take a moment to reflect on your progress. Check off all you've added to your routine:

- ❑ Are you taking a daily forty-five-minute walk?
- ❑ Are you working in frequent exercise snacks?
- ❑ Have you added a weekly strength-training session?
- ❑ Are you continuing to minimize blue-light exposure at night?
- ❑ Are you viewing sunlight as soon as you wake up?
- ❑ Are you eating balanced meals with enough calories, using the best carbs, fats, and proteins at the right macronutrient ratios?

Embrace these new challenges with enthusiasm, knowing that your future self will be so thankful you made these changes. As you incorporate these habits, keep in mind that consistency is key. Commit to your walking time, exercise snacks, and weekly strength training. Trust the process. Your body will adapt and grow stronger with each passing day, and the benefits will extend far beyond the physical realm. As your cells produce energy more efficiently, you'll likely feel sharper. You may also handle stress better and feel healthier overall.

Week 4: Boost Your Movement and Reassess Progress

Let's kick things up a notch in week 4. You've been doing great with your exercise snacks, but now it's time to amplify your efforts. Continue incorporating those unlimited exercise snacks throughout your day, but also increase your thirty-minute strength training to twice weekly. Focus on fundamental movements like squatting, pushing, and pulling. These compound exercises engage multiple muscle groups simultaneously, maximizing your workout efficiency and promoting overall strength gains.

As you progress, challenge your muscles by gradually increasing the weight or resistance. This concept, known as progressive overload, is the key to continuous improvement. But don't sacrifice form for weight. Maintaining proper technique and focusing on the correct working muscle is crucial for preventing injuries and ensuring you reap the full benefits of each exercise. Listen to your body and adjust as needed. Remember, consistency trumps intensity every time.

This week you also need to reassess your metabolic rate. By now, you've likely noticed some positive changes in your digestion and overall well-being. It's time to take a closer look at how your body has responded to the dietary changes you've implemented. If you've been using the Food Buddy app or keeping a food journal, review your entries. Look for patterns or correlations between your food choices and your energy levels, mood, sleep quality, and digestive comfort. This information is gold. It's your body communicating with you, telling you what works and what doesn't.

To gauge your metabolic progress, recheck your body temperature. Take measurements immediately upon waking, forty minutes after breakfast, and again forty minutes after lunch for a few days this week. Compare these to your week 1 measurements. You should see a rise in your body temperature, indicating that your metabolism is revving up. This is a fantastic sign! It means your body now has access to more cellular energy, allowing it to reactivate functions that may have been suppressed due to a slower metabolic rate.

If you're not seeing the temperature increase you hoped for, don't worry. Metabolism healing is not always a rapid process. Patience and persistence are key. Here are some tweaks to boost your body temperature (and thus your metabolic rate):

- Ensure you're eating a substantial breakfast to kick-start heat production early in the day. Reduce your consumption of cold foods and drinks. Opt for room-temperature or warmer choices instead.

- Eat every three to six hours to keep your metabolism humming and reduce stress responses.

- Make sure you're consuming enough calories and carbohydrates. Chronic undereating will hinder energy production.

- Find ways to lower stress in your life and engage in a creative activity you enjoy for at least five minutes daily. This could be anything from singing to drawing to spending time with loved ones—whatever helps you enter a relaxed, parasympathetic state.

Next, assess your gut health. If you've been following the Metabolic Boost program from week 2, it's time to check your progress. Are you having one to three bowel movements daily? Do you feel energized and mentally clear?

Has your gut discomfort and distress diminished or disappeared? If you answered yes to these questions, congratulations! You're on the right track. If not, don't be discouraged. Improving systemic energy production takes time. Ensure you're consuming enough calories: anything under 1,800 calories daily can hinder metabolic improvement. Ideally aim for 2,000 calories or more without weight gain.

It's also time to introduce a wider variety of foods, particularly carbohydrates. Add new foods one at a time, paying close attention to how your body responds. If you notice any adverse reactions, make a note and avoid that food for now. If your body tolerates it well, incorporate it into your regular meal rotation. Remember, the ability to tolerate a wide variety of foods is a sign of good health. Starches are particularly important for supporting mitochondrial energy production, so don't shy away from potatoes, rice, and other healthy carbs.

As week 4 ends, take a moment to reassess your caloric needs. Note any weight changes from your baseline. While it's okay to want to lose weight, it's much easier to do so with a well-functioning metabolism. Prioritize improving your metabolic rate first, which will make future weight-loss efforts more effective and sustainable. Remember, weight-loss phases should be limited to two to three months to prevent metabolic downregulation.

Week 4 Checklist

- ❑ Are you taking a daily one-hour walk, continuing to avoid solar noon until you've been off seed oils for six months?

- ❑ Are you continuing to incorporate exercise snacks throughout the day?

- ❑ Are you minimizing blue-light exposure at night?

- ❑ Are you viewing the sun or horizon upon waking to optimize your circadian rhythm?

- ❑ Are you eating balanced meals with sufficient calories?

- ❑ Are you completing two 30-minute strength-training sessions weekly?

- ❑ Have you experimented with adding foods back into your diet?

- ❑ Have you monitored your body temperature as a gauge of your progress? Remember to aim for a waking temperature in the high 97°F range, rising to 98.6°F by midday, as this is a clear sign of optimal energy production.

- ❑ Are you committed to continuing to use the free Mercola Health Coach app beyond this four-week program?

As you wrap up the four weeks, take time to reflect on your progress. Notice how your energy levels have changed, how your sleep has improved, and how your body feels. These changes attest to the power of diet, exercise, and lifestyle in boosting your metabolism.

But remember, your journey doesn't end here. The habits you've developed over these four weeks form the foundation for long-term metabolic health. Continue to listen to your body, adjust as needed, and celebrate your progress along the way. Also remember that this program is always here if you need a reset in the future.

Scan this QR code to get FREE access to the Mercola Health Coach app. This tool allows you to log your meals, track your macronutrient ratios, and monitor your progress over time.

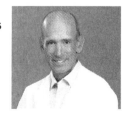

CHAPTER 13

Nurturing Your Cellular Vitality in Today's World

Since the biologist and conservationist Rachel Carson's *Silent Spring*, we've faced many new environmental threats. Today, we're battling a complex web of interrelated health hazards that Carson could scarcely have imagined. Three modern pollutants are especially harmful: vegetable and seed oils, electromagnetic fields (EMFs), and microplastics.

A century ago, vegetable and seed oils made up less than 2 percent of the average diet. Today? A staggering 19–22 percent. This isn't just a change in your menu; it's a fundamental shift in your body's biochemistry. These oils have disrupted your metabolism and gut bacteria. They are behind the rise in chronic diseases, making obesity, diabetes, and other metabolic disorders societal issues—not to mention the effect the increase in these illnesses has had on our health-care systems.

Then there's the invisible threat of EMFs. Your cell phones, Wi-Fi routers, and other electronic devices are bathing you in a sea of radiation. Research shows a link between EMF exposure, sleep issues, and DNA damage. It paints a disturbing picture of our tech-saturated world. I've seen patients whose health improved after making "EMF-free" zones in their homes, especially in their bedrooms.

But perhaps most alarming is our regular consumption of microplastics. Did you know you're ingesting the equivalent of a credit card's worth of plastic each week? These tiny particles carry xenoestrogens that radically disrupt your endocrine system. The scope of this threat is staggering, infiltrating your body through food, water, and even the air you breathe.

At the heart of all these issues are your mitochondria. They are your cellular powerhouses and defenders against modern pollutants. Mitochondrial dysfunction isn't just a curiosity but the key to disease. The core issue is a lack of cellular energy, which is needed to fuel your biology and activate your natural repair and regeneration pathways. These environmental assaults have harmed your cells, which then produce less energy, causing your health crisis.

Despite all these factors, there is reason for hope. Just as Carson's work sparked a revolution in environmental awareness, your knowledge can now fuel change. You have the power to make informed choices about your diet, technology use, and consumption habits. You can demand better from policymakers and industries.

The path forward requires a holistic, integrated approach. You need to reimagine your relationship with the world around you. Focus on whole, unprocessed foods over those containing harmful industrial oils. Create EMF-free zones in your home. Radically reduce your use of plastic products. On a broader scale, support research into safer alternatives. Advocate for stricter rules on endocrine-disrupting chemicals and push for more sustainable food production methods. Your health and the health of our planet depend on it.

Empowering Your Health Journey: From Knowledge to Action

The key to turning this ship around? Education. We need to spread awareness about mitochondrial health like it's our job—because in a way, it is. Your mitochondria are your cells' powerhouses. If they fail, chaos ensues. I've seen so many patients change their lives for the better by understanding how their cellular energy affects their health.

But this is not easy. There are many competing influences that seek to intentionally deceive and confuse you. As you navigate this complex landscape, you must remain open to new information. The field of health is constantly evolving, and what we know today might be refined tomorrow.

The challenges we collectively face may seem daunting. But let me tell you, they're not insurmountable. By understanding these threats, you're already better equipped to navigate them. You have the knowledge and tools to make a difference—use them!

It's time to reclaim and take control of your health, protect the environment, and create a better world for future generations. This isn't just about you—it's about all of us and the planet we call home. Make conscious choices in your daily life. Advocate for change on a larger scale. Reconnect with the natural world. Remember, when you protect your health, you're also safeguarding the health of the planet.

The time to act is now. We need to heed the lessons of the past, confront our present challenges, and work together for a harmonious future. But you don't have to do this alone. I've developed resources to support you on this journey.

The Mercola Health Coach app—which is free on iOS and Android—helps you track your progress, set health goals, and receive personalized advice. If you'd like more in-depth guidance, we offer virtual health-coach consultations. These one-on-one sessions let you address specific concerns. They also let you tailor your approach to cellular healing.

For affordable access to specialized testing and in-person support from health experts trained in the concepts in this book, Mercola Health Clinics provide hands-on support, specialized testing, and access to health experts. Because the path to better health begins with informed, consistent choices, we are working hard to give you multiple ways to gain access to information and expertise that help you consistently make those choices. As mentioned in the introduction to this book, health-care providers in the US write over six billion prescriptions annually, which breaks down to 17 prescriptions per person each year. Chances are, you are currently taking one or more medications yourself. To address this, our team of health coaches includes trained and licensed doctors of pharmacy who, instead of filling prescriptions, now work to help get people off drugs.

As we wrap up, I want to encourage you to stay curious, stay informed, and stay committed to making positive changes. The power to transform your health at a cellular level is in your hands. We've provided the information and support system—now it's up to you to take the first step on this journey toward vibrant, energetic living. Trust me, it's a journey worth taking.

Remember, you're not just changing your habits; you're unlocking your body's potential and joining a health-care revolution. By combining cutting-edge technology with a deep understanding of cellular energy and metabolic health, you are part of a paradigm shift in wellness. Your dedication and willingness to challenge the status quo are driving this movement forward. Together, we're building a community of empowered individuals, supporting and inspiring each other on this journey to optimal health.

Let's step boldly into a future of boundless health, vitality, and Joy.

Scan this QR code to get FREE access to the Mercola Health Coach app. This tool allows you to log your meals, track your macronutrient ratios, and monitor your progress over time.

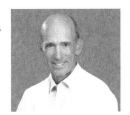

REFERENCES

Unparalleled Scientific Backing

 One of the major strengths of this book is its extensive and up-to-date scientific foundation. It contains 2,500 references, with the majority sourced from studies conducted in the 2020s. Over 95 percent of these citations include direct links to the full-text scientific papers. This level of accessibility allows you the opportunity to directly explore the primary science for yourself. You can verify any claims and expand your understanding beyond the book's content.

By providing links to original research, I hope to empower you to critically evaluate the information presented. This approach aligns with the scientific method. It allows you to examine evidence first-hand rather than relying solely on the interpretation. This approach allows a facilitated and more nuanced understanding of the topics discussed and enables you to form your own evidence-based conclusions.

It's important to understand that this book is not the definitive answer to optimizing your biology and health. Science is constantly evolving, and our understanding of health continues to be refined with new research. This is why we need a dynamic system that can access and interpret scientific literature in real time, allowing us to continuously update our knowledge and recommendations. Our upcoming Mercola Health Coach system is designed to contribute to this ongoing process by collecting valuable data.

In the future, we aim to publish hundreds of articles based on this data and emerging research. These publications will help to further refine our understanding of how to effectively optimize cellular energy production and overall health. Our goal is to create a continuously evolving body of knowledge that adapts to the latest scientific discoveries, ensuring that you always have access to the most current and accurate information to make informed decisions about your health.

INDEX